ENDOCRINOLOGY RESEARCH AND CLINICAL DEVELOPMENTS

ENDOCRINE DISEASES

RISK FACTORS, DIAGNOSIS AND MANAGEMENT

ENDOCRINOLOGY RESEARCH AND CLINICAL DEVELOPMENTS

Additional books in this series can be found on Nova's website
under the Series tab.

Additional e-books in this series can be found on Nova's website
under the e-book tab.

ENDOCRINOLOGY RESEARCH AND CLINICAL DEVELOPMENTS

ENDOCRINE DISEASES

RISK FACTORS, DIAGNOSIS AND MANAGEMENT

KENNETH HINES
EDITOR

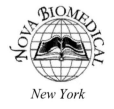

Nova Biomedical

New York

We have partnered with Copyright Clearance Center to make it easy for you to obtain permissions to reuse content from this publication. Simply navigate to this publication's page on Nova's website and locate the "Get Permission" button below the title description. This button is linked directly to the title's permission page on copyright.com. Alternatively, you can visit copyright.com and search by title, ISBN, or ISSN.

For further questions about using the service on copyright.com, please contact:
Copyright Clearance Center
Phone: +1-(978) 750-8400   Fax: +1-(978) 750-4470   E-mail: info@copyright.com.

NOTICE TO THE READER

The Publisher has taken reasonable care in the preparation of this book, but makes no expressed or implied warranty of any kind and assumes no responsibility for any errors or omissions. No liability is assumed for incidental or consequential damages in connection with or arising out of information contained in this book. The Publisher shall not be liable for any special, consequential, or exemplary damages resulting, in whole or in part, from the readers' use of, or reliance upon, this material. Any parts of this book based on government reports are so indicated and copyright is claimed for those parts to the extent applicable to compilations of such works.

Independent verification should be sought for any data, advice or recommendations contained in this book. In addition, no responsibility is assumed by the publisher for any injury and/or damage to persons or property arising from any methods, products, instructions, ideas or otherwise contained in this publication.

This publication is designed to provide accurate and authoritative information with regard to the subject matter covered herein. It is sold with the clear understanding that the Publisher is not engaged in rendering legal or any other professional services. If legal or any other expert assistance is required, the services of a competent person should be sought. FROM A DECLARATION OF PARTICIPANTS JOINTLY ADOPTED BY A COMMITTEE OF THE AMERICAN BAR ASSOCIATION AND A COMMITTEE OF PUBLISHERS.

Additional color graphics may be available in the e-book version of this book.

Library of Congress Cataloging-in-Publication Data

ISBN: 978-1-63482-592-4
Library of Congress Control Number: 2015940902

Published by Nova Science Publishers, Inc. † New York

Contents

Preface

The human body's endocrine system includes eight major glands, which make hormones and travel through the bloodstream to tissues or organs. In this book, the authors' focus on the risk factors, genetics, diagnosis and management of gynecomastia (a benign condition characterized by enlargement of the male breast) and addresses the puzzling controversies surrounding menopausal hormone replacement therapy (HRT) and its health outcomes, which have been the subject of extensive investigation in recent years. The book concludes with a bibliography on recent titles published in the field that readers might find of interest.

Chapter 1 – The term gynecomastia was coined by the Roman physician Claudius Galenus (129-200 AD) and refers to a benign condition characterized by enlargement of the male breast, which can be physically uncomfortable, psychologically distressing, and may have a negative impact on self-confidence and body image. Pseudogynecomastia is common in obese men, and consists of fat deposition, without glandular proliferation. Most of gynecomastia treated by surgeons is mixed, with both glandular proliferation and fat deposition.

Chapter 2 – Gynecomastia is a benign disease defined by enlargement of the male mammary gland. Dysregulation of the androgen-estrogen balance is the main underlying mechanism. The most common form of this disease is the physiologic gynecomastia, caused by normal transient or permanent changes. It is characterized by three peaks of prevalence at the neonatal, pubertal, and adult period. The neonatal gynecomastia is transient and resolves within a year, while the underlying cause is the maternal-placental estrogens, which circulate in the neonate. The pubertal gynecomastia is transient and resolves within two years. The underlying cause is an estrogen increase due to testicular stimulation by gonadotrophins. The adult gynecomastia is observed mainly in men aged 50 to 80 years and it is correlated with physiologic changes of aged-related change, such as a decline in androgen levels, increase of adipose tissue and increased aromatase activity resulting in an upregulation of circulating estrogens. However, except from the physiologic causes of gynecomastia there are also pathologic ones covering a wide range of different diseases. The pathologic gynecomastia affects men in any age and does not follow the three peaks pattern of prevalence observed at the physiologic form. The pathologic reasons can be divided into three categories: a) systemic diseases comprising tumors producing hormones and chronic diseases of liver and kidneys. b) Endocrinological diseases including thyroid, adrenal, gonadal, and pituitary dysfunction. c) Iatrogenic causes and exogenous agents, which develop into gynecomastia through different mechanisms, such as direct action of estrogens or estrogen-like substances and inhibition of androgen production or androgen receptor's function. These agents are pharmaceutical substances used for diseases such as hypertension, congestive heart failure, HIV infection, gastroesophageal reflux disease, benign prostate hyperplasia and prostate cancer. Gynecomastia has a strong genetic background. It is developed in several disorders of sexual hormones or organs derived from chromosomal anomalies, gene mutations, and polymorphisms. Common syndromes such as Klinefelter's and Peutz-Jeghers as well as rare syndromes such as Borjeson-Forssman-Lehmann are described to have gynecomastia as one of the characteristic anomalies. Other disorders related to gynecomastia are the aromatase excess syndrome, Kennedy's disease, and androgen insensitivity syndrome. Finally, there are polymorphisms in genes such as *CYP19, ERS2,* and *LEPR,* which are shown to be the causative factor of gynectomastia.

Gynecomastia is considered a benign disorder without a strong correlation with breast cancer, except in the case of Klinefelter's syndrome. The cause of pathologic gynecomastia could vary from the administration of an exogenous agent to the polymorphism of a single gene. Therefore, males should be examined and investigated for a causative factor with great attention especially when gynecomastia is accompanied with infertility.

Chapter 3 – Menopausal hormone replacement therapy (HRT) and its health outcomes have been the subjects of extensive investigation; the results of these however are highly inconclusive. Today, it is considered that the effect of HRT is a complex pattern of the mysterious mixture of risks and benefits and the use of this therapy is not evaluated as safety prevention for chronic diseases. This conclusion implies the unawareness of the crucial role of estrogens in the surveillance of cellular health based on the misinterpretation of clinical and experimental results. Estrogens and their receptor system have biologically pivotal role favored by evolution as a means of integration of all cellular functions serving the survival and reproduction of individuals. A unique feature of estrogens is their beneficial safeguard on all privileged healthy cells, while they are capable of recognizing malignant tumor cells and killing them by apoptosis. All previous studies related to women receiving HRT were performed on randomly selected patients, disregarding their risk factors for either insufficient estrogen synthesis or defective estrogen receptor transduction pathways. Recently, the Women's Health Initiative (WHI) Randomized Trials, which examined the effect of HRT on hysterectomised, crudely estrogen deficient women, found that estrogen treatment resulted in striking decreases in breast cancer development. Moreover, after re-analyzing the data of earlier WHI studies, subsets of women without strong family history of breast cancer, exhibited significantly reduced breast cancer incidence attributable to one armed estrogen treatment. At the same time, women with a family history of breast cancer could have inherited defective estrogen receptor signaling and reactive but insufficient hyperestrogenism. The perspectives for successful HRT will be the separation of postmenopausal patients according to their different inclination to breast cancer risk. The appropriate estrogen dosage will be beneficial against breast cancer and for many other aspects of women's health as well.

In: Endocrine Diseases
Editor: Kenneth Hines

ISBN: 978-1-63482-592-4
© 2015 Nova Science Publishers, Inc.

Chapter 1

Gynecomastia: Risk Factors, Diagnosis and Management

Jesús Benito-Ruiz and Marisa Manzano*

Department of Plastic Surgery, Clinica Tres Torres, Barcelona, Spain

The term gynecomastia was coined by the Roman physician Claudius Galenus (129-200 AD) [1] and refers to a benign condition characterized by enlargement of the male breast, which can be physically uncomfortable, psychologically distressing, and may have a negative impact on self-confidence and body image. Pseudogynecomastia is common in obese men, and consists of fat deposition, without glandular proliferation. Most of gynecomastia treated by surgeons is mixed, with both glandular proliferation and fat deposition [2].

Sixty to ninety percent of male infants have neonatal gynecomastia due to high estrogen state during pregnancy. During pregnancy, the placenta converts DHEA (dehydroepiandrosterone) and DHEA-SO4 (dehydroepiandrosterone-sulfate), derived from both mother and fetus, to estrone and estradiol, respectively. Estrone and estradiol then enters the fetal circulation and stimulates breast glandular proliferation. Pubertal gynecomastia has a peak prevalence of nearly 65%, starting at 12 yrs of age, and with a peak at about 14

---

* Address: Dr. Jesús Benito-Ruiz, c/ Dr. Carulla 12, 3rd floor, 08017 Barcelona. drbenito@ antiaginggroupbarcelona.com.

years of age. Older men also develop involutional gynecomastia, with a prevalence of 40-55%, linked to increase in adiposity and decrease in testosterone [3, 4].

The clinical aspects of gynecomastia are [5]:

- an increase in the areolar diameter;
- breast swelling, altering the profile of the male thorax;
- anomalous presence of an inframammary fold;
- cutaneous ptosis with the nipple-areola complex sliding down to the height of the fold or even below it;
- asymmetry

Several morphological classifications have been reported depending on skin elasticity, volume, the presence of an inframammary fold, mammary ptosis, or the relationship between the nipple-areola complex and the inframammary fold. The main used classifications for gynecomastia are resumed in Table 1. [2, 5-8]

Histology

Gynecomastia at its early stages is characterized by ductal epithelial hyperplasia (the proliferation and lengthening of the ducts), an increase in stromal and periductal connective tissue, increased periductal inflammation, intensive periductal edema, and stromal fibroblastic proliferation. Pain or tenderness is common in the beginning, but it disappears in later stages (after 12m), where there is marked stromal fibrosis, a slight increase in the number of ducts, but little to no epithelial proliferation, and no inflammatory response [9]. Medical treatment can therefore be beneficial if implemented during the early proliferative phase, before the glandular structure has been replaced by stromal hyalinization and fibrosis [2].

Physiopathology

The altered ratio of estrogens to androgens or increased breast sensitivity to normal circulating estrogen levels results in ductal hyperplasia, elongation, and branching, along with fibroblast proliferation and increased vascularity [7-

10]. Estrogen in men comes primarily from converting peripheral androgens, testosterone and rostenedione, to estradiol and estrone via the aromatase enzyme. This occurs mainly in muscle, fat, and skin. [4, 10-12].

Table 1.

Barros [2] Cordova [5]	Ratnam [6]	Simon [7]	Rohrich [8]
increase in diameter and protrusion limited to the areolar region	enlarged breasts with elastic skin and no fold;	Grade I: Small enlargement without skin excess	Minimal hypertrophy (< 250 g) without ptosis
hypertrophy of all the structural components of the breast. The nipple-areola complex is above the inframammary fold	enlarged breasts with elastic skin and an IM	Grade IIa: Moderate enlargement without skin excess	Moderate hypertrophy (250–500 g) without ptosis
hypertrophy of all the structural components, nipple-areola complex at the same height as or about 1 cm below the inframammary fold; in this group we can also include male tuberous breast	ptotic breasts with inelastic skin	Grade IIb: Moderate enlargement with minor skin excess	Severe hypertrophy (> 500 g) with grade I ptosis
hypertrophy of all the structural components, nipple-areola complex more than 1 cm below the inframammary fold		Grade III: Marked enlargement with excess skin, mimicking female breast ptosis	Severe hypertrophy with grade II or grade III ptosis

The estrogen/androgen imbalance may be attributable to internal causes (increased secretion of estrogens by the testes or adrenal glands, extra glandular aromatization of estrogen precursors, decreased estrogen degradation) or external, such as exposure to estrogen-like chemicals, or exogenous estrogens and use of drugs [13].

On the other side, the imbalance may result from decreased androgen production in the testes, increased binding of androgens (relative to estrogens) by Sex Hormone Binding Globuline, altered androgen metabolism, drug-induced displacement of androgens from their receptors and androgen receptor defects. [4, 13]

Table 2.

Physiologic	Pathologic	Medication
Neonatal Pubertal Involutional	*Neoplasms* • Testicular • Pituitary • Breast tumors • Adrenal • Liver • Human Chorionic Gonadotropin-ectopic production • Lymphoma/leukemia *Endocrinopathies* • Hypogonadism • Syndromes: Klinefelter, Kallman's • Androgen insensitivity • Hermaphroditism • Enzymatic defects of testosterone synthesis • Testicular injury/regression • Hyperthyroidism • High aromatase • Adrenal hyperplasia • Corticotropin deficiency *Chronic Illnesses* • Liver disease • Renal disease • Malnutrition • Cystic fibrosis • AIDS • Ulcerative Colitis	*Hormones* • Estrogens and estrogen agonists • Androgens and anabolic steroids • Human chorionic gonadotropin *Androgen antagonists* • Ketoconazole • Flutamide • Metronidazole • Finasteride • Spironolactone • Etomidate *Antiulcer drugs* • Cimetidine • Omeprazole • Ranitidine *Cytotoxic agents* • Bisulfar • Vincristine • Nitrosoureas • Procarbazine • Cisplatin • Methotrexate • Cyclophosphamide • Chlorambucil *Psychoactive drugs* • Tricyclic antidepressants • Phenothiazines • Diazepam *Cardiovascular agents* • Amiodarone • Angiotensin-converting enzyme inhibitors • Calcium channel blockers • Digitoxin • Methyldopa

Physiologic	Pathologic	Medication
		Antituberculotic agents • Ethionamide • Thiacetazone • Isoniazid *Antiviral therapeutics* • Protease inhibiters *Miscellaneous* • Marijuana • Heroine • Methadone • Alcohol • Amphetamines • Phenytoin • Penicillamine

Another hormonal action that stimulates breast tissue in men is observed secondary to hyperprolactinemia. Prolactin receptors have been demonstrated in gynecomastia, but it does not seem that it is an important cause for gynecomastia, because most men with gynecomastia do not have elevated serum prolactin levels and not all men with hyperprolactinemia develop gynecomastia [3].

Causes of Gynecomastia

The incidence of the different etiologies for gynecomastia is as follows [14]:

- Idiopathic gynecomastia (no detectable abnormality) 25%
- Pubertal gynecomastia 25%
- Secondary to medication 10–20%
- Cirrhosis or malnutrition 8%
- Primary hypogonadism 8%
- Testicular tumors 3%
- Secondary hypogonadism 2%
- Hyperthyroidism 1.5%
- Chronic renal disease 1%

In our practice, 70% of patients have either idiopathic or pubertal gynecomastia (many of them who suffer are adults with gynecomastia since their puberty). 20% are due to intake of anabolic steroids and 10% are involutional (senile) gynecomastia.

Pubertal gynecomastia is so far the most common. It appears to be due to an elevated conversion of adrenal androgens to estrogens during daytime when testosterone secretion is low (in puberty testosterone usually is secreted at night) [15]. In 75% of teenagers with gynecomastia, this disappears in 2-3 years after onset.

The main causes for gynecomastia [14] are summarized in Table 2.

Evaluation

Most of patients present to the surgeon after being evaluated by an endocrinologist. If this has not been so, medical evaluation should include [3, 14]:

- Detailed family history and medical history to identify any of the causes listed above, especially cirrhosis, renal failure, hyperthyroidism, medication.
- Physical exploration of abdomen and testes
- Laboratory assessment for renal, hepatic and thyroid function
- Mainly in boys, Luteinizing hormone, follicule-stimulating hormone, estradiol, dehydroepiandrosterone and chorionic gonadotropin.
- Mammogram and ultrasonography are not strictly necessary, but they can be useful especially in senile gynecomastia for differential diagnosis of breast cancer, and especially if the patient has breast discharge, bleeding, unilateral gynecomastia, or skin dimpling [16]. Frazier [17] distinguishes three patterns of gynecomastia in mammographies: Florid (large, irregular, subareolar density), Dendritic (smaller, speculated, subareola density and extensive stromal fibrosis) and Diffuse (mimics the heterogeneously female breast). Ultrasonography is also helpful to differentiate true gynecomastia from pseudogynecomastia and is useful to decide the best surgical technique.

The main clinical differences between breast cancer and gynecomastia are [18]:

Gynecomastia	Breast Cancer
Bilateral (usually) or unilateral	Unilateral (usually) or bilateral
Painless or painful (occasionally)	Painless or painful (uncommon)
Central (subareolar)	Central (70-90%) or eccentric
Smooth	Irregular
Firm	Rubbery or hard
Mobile	Fixed
Normal nipple	Nipple deformity (17-30%) or discharge (< 10%)
Normal skin	Thickened, red, or ulcerated skin
Normal axilla	Axillary adenopathy

Medical Treatment

Antiestrogens (tamoxifen and raloxifene) have been used to decrease the effects of estrogens on the male breast and treat the gynecomastia [19-24]. Tamoxifen has been used in doses of 10-20 mg/day and raloxifene at 60 mg/day, for 3-9 months. In Parker's et al. study [19], one-month courses of a placebo or the antiestrogen tamoxifen (10 mg given orally bid) were compared in random order. Seven of ten patients experienced a decrease in the size of their gynecomastia due to tamoxifen (P less than 0.005). Overall, the decrease for gynecomastia was significant for the whole group (P less than 0.01). There was no beneficial effect of placebo (P greater than 0.1). Additionally, all four patients with painful gynecomastia experienced symptomatic relief. There was no toxicity.

Lawrence et al. [20] studied the efficacy of both tamoxifen and raloxifen in 38 patients with pubertal gynecomastia. Mean (SD) age of treated subjects was 14.6 (1.5) years with gynecomastia duration of 28.3 (16.4) months. Mean reduction in breast nodule diameter was 2.1 cm (95% CI 1.7, 2.7, P <.0001) after treatment with tamoxifen, and 2.5 cm (95% CI 1.7, 3.3, P <.0001) with raloxifene. Some improvement was seen in 86% of patients receiving tamoxifen and in 91% receiving raloxifene, but a greater proportion had a significant decrease (> 50%) with raloxifene (86%) than tamoxifen (41%). No side effects were seen in any patients.

In the study by Khan et al. [22], thirty-six men were treated with tamoxifen for physiological gynecomastia. Median age was 31 (range 18-64). Tenderness was present in 25 (71%) cases. Sixteen men (45%) had 'fatty' gynecomastia and 20 had 'lump' gynecomastia. Tamoxifen resolved the mass in 30 patients (83.3%; CR = 22, PR = 8) and tenderness in 21 cases (84%; CR = 0, PR = 0). Lump gynecomastia was more responsive to tamoxifen than the fatty type (100% vs. 62.5%; P = 0.0041).

Devoto et al. [24] treated forty three patients with gynecomastia, aged 12 to 62 years. Twenty patients had mastodynia and in 33, gynecomastia had a diameter over 4 cm. It lasted less than two years in 30 patients, more than two years in nine, and four did not recall its duration. All were treated with tamoxifen 20 mg/day for 6 months. Mastodynia disappeared in all patients at three months. At six months gynecomastia disappeared in 26 patients (62%), but relapsed in 27%. All gynecomastias caused by drugs with antiandrogen activity disappeared. Fifty two percent of gynecomastias over 4 cm and 90% of those of less than 4 cm in diameter disappeared (p<0.05). Fifty-six percent of gynecomastias lasted more than two years and 70% of those of a shorter duration disappeared.

Anastrozol, an aromatase inhibitor, has also been studied for the treatment of gynecomastia. It seems that it has not been as effective as tamoxifen for breast reduction [25].

Surgical Treatment

The first reported surgical treatment of gynecomastia was by Paulus Aegineta (625-690 AD), who used a lunate incision below the breast or, for larger breasts, two converging lunate incisions to enable the excision of excess skin [26]. In the Islamic world, Abulcasis (Al-Zahrawi) in Cordoba, Spain, described two different surgical techniques for the treatment of gynecomastia. The first technique included making a lunate incision above the breast, removal of the subcutaneous fat, and application of a cicatrizing compound. In contrast to the site of incision (below the breast) indicated by Paulus of Aegina, Al-Zahrawi recommended making the incision above the breast. The second surgical technique, described by Al-Zahrawi for the treatment of gynecomastia, involved making two lunate incisions along the upper part of the breast to allow the removal of subcutaneous fat and redundant skin as well as application of styptic powder. Al-Zahrawi indicated hemorrhage as a complication of the surgical management of gynecomastia and, therefore, he recommended compression cotton dressing [1].

In 1946, Webster was the first to abandon extra-areolar skin incisions in favor of a semicircular intra-areolar incision [27]. This approach has been the gold standard for years for the surgical treatment of gynecomastia.

The objectives of surgical treatment are [5]:

- flattening of the thoracic region;
- elimination of the inframammary fold;
- correct positioning of the nipple-areola complex;
- removal of redundant skin;
- symmetrization between the two hemithoraxes and the two areolas;
- containment of scars.

Controversy arises when surgical treatment is indicated in the pubertal age. Traditionally, it has been recommended to wait until the spontaneous regression of the breast enlargement. However, gynecomastia can be quite distressing at this age and recent papers recommend early surgical treatment to avoid the unwanted psychological sequelae [28, 29]. Adolescent boys with this condition frequently experience significant psychosocial problems because of the gender-incongruent appearance of their chests, including low self-esteem, body-image disturbances, and teasing related to breast enlargement. Many affected adolescent boys camouflage the appearance of their chests by wearing loose or oversized shirts or binding their chests with tape or other restrictive materials. They may avoid situations and activities in which their chest may be exposed [30].

A significant step forward in the treatment of gynecomastia was with the introduction of liposuction by Illouz in the late 1970s [31], as it enabled the contouring of enlarged breasts through very small incisions. In the late 1980s, Zocchi developed ultrasound-assisted liposuction, a technique that allows selective destruction of adipose tissue [32]. Liposuction is very effective to remove the fatty component of the gynecomastia, but not for the fibroglandular tissue. Several techniques have been reported to excise the glandular tissue once the fat has been removed with liposuction, such as ultrasound [8, 26, 33, 34], laser [35, 36], pull-through [37, 38], radio frequency [39], cutting cannulas [40] or cartilage shavers [41].

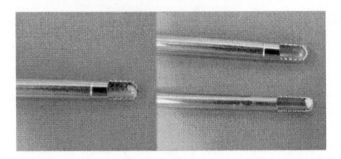

Figure 1. Close up view of the tip of the arthroscopic shaver (called full radius).

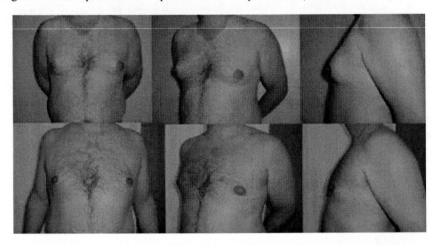

Figure 2. A 32 year old male patient with grade II gynecomastia treated with de Prado's technique. Preoperative (above) and postoperative views (below) at 12 months.

In severe cases (grade III and IV) skin excision techniques might be necessary. The main problem with these procedures is the scar, which could be an important sequela itself. Skin can be removed around the areola [42, 43], or through a horizontal excision, leaving the nipple areola complex on a dermal pedicle [44].

Our preferred method for correcting gynecomastia is De Prado's technique [41, 45, 46]. Our surgical technique is as follows [45]:

The patient is marked preoperatively standing upright. All patients are treated under general anesthesia. The patient was placed in a supine position on the operating table with his arms abducted at 90°. The entire surgical area is infiltrated with a wetting solution through a stab incision located inferolaterally. First of all, a conventional liposuction is performed using a 3 or 4 mm cannula. To remove the gland a suction assisted cartilage shaver (Striker

Endoscopic Arthroscopic System SE 5/TPS) is used. The blade is comprised of two concentric cannulas with diameters of 3 and 4 mm. The outer cannula has an upward opening hub with a grid to allow the rotating inner cannula to serve as a continuous curette (Figure 1). The inner cannula rotates in oscillation mode. With back and forth movements the tissue is severed and suctioned. It is very important to leave a small amount of gland behind the areola to avoid antiaesthetic depression. Homogeneity and regularity were determined using the pinch test. The non-dominant hand tells the surgeon how much gland to remove, controlling the thickness of the flap (video). Care must be exerted to avoid curetting the dermis. When the procedure was completed, we sutured the small incisions and applied sterile, compressive dressing. The patient is discharged the day after surgery.

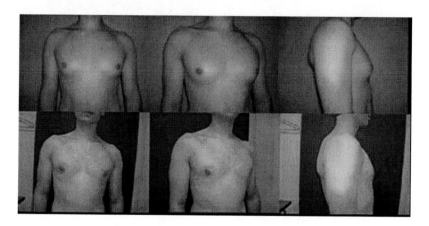

Figure 3. A 22-year-old male patient with grade II gynecomastia treated with de Prado's technique. Preoperative (above) and postoperative views (below) at 8 months.

This technique is mainly indicated for grades II and III (Figures 2-6). We performed this operation in 40 consecutive cases with different degrees of severity and we conclude that it is not suitable for patients with Grade I (just sub areolar, glandular enlargement and no fat). The risk for problems (irregularities, skin pigmentation) is quite high. In these patients we prefer the classic areolar approach (Figure 7) or a mastectomy through the axilla (usually endoscopic) (Figures 8-10). For the axillary approach we first detach the fibroglandular tissue from the skin and we leave a small subareolar patch to avoid skin retraction. The second step is to detach the posterior aspect of the gland with a subfascial technique. Finally we have to cut the most caudal aspect, which is usually the most demanding step and the entire piece is removed through the incision (Figure 11).

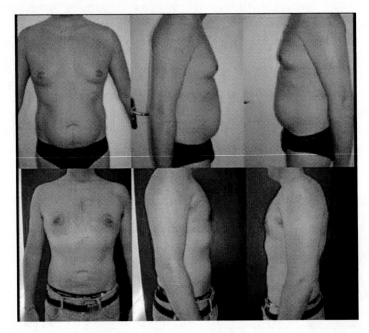

Figure 4. A 29-year-old male patient with grade II gynecomastia treated with de Prado's technique and abdominal liposuction. Preoperative (above) and postoperative views (below) at 12 months. Some patients benefit from a combined approach treating chest and abdomen as an entire aesthetic unit.

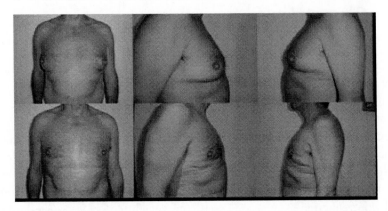

Figure 5. A 62-year-old male patient with grade III gynecomastia treated with de Prado's technique. Preoperative (above) and postoperative views (below) at 6 months.

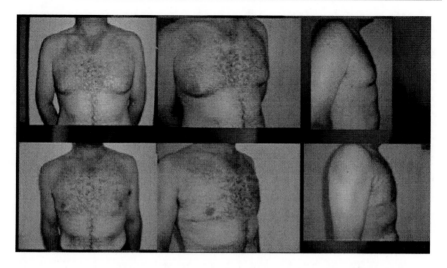

Figure 6. A 32-year-old male patient with grade II gynecomastia treated with de Prado's technique. Preoperative (above) and postoperative views (below) at 6 months.

Unless we face a very severe problem with the skin excess, we prefer to reduce volume with liposuction as a first step and wait one year for the skin shrinkage. After this time, the patient is reevaluated to decide if skin excision is necessary (Figure 12). However, sometimes it is unavoidable to perform direct skin excision in the first procedure, because of the ptosis and volume that the breasts have (Figures 13 and 14).

The main complications in surgical management of gynecomastia are:

- Hematoma: expansive hematoma could lead to nipple areola necrosis or to fibrosis and skin irregularities.
- Excessive excision leaving to areolar depression and irregularities (Figure 15)
- Incomplete excision (Figure 16)
- Skin hyperpigmentation

Hematoma is probably the most common complication reported, around 4% [8, 47]. Our rate of hematoma requiring reoperation is zero so far. To prevent hematoma we always use a compressive bandage for 24 hours. It is then substituted by a compressive garment to be worn all day for one month. Gentle massaging on the operated area is advised after the first 48 hours.

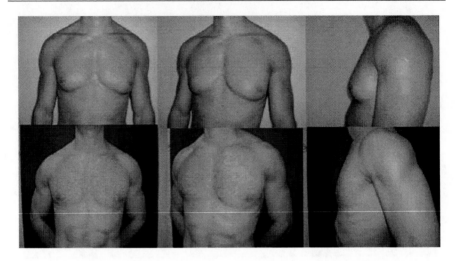

Figure 7. A 23-year-old male patient with gynecomastia due to anabolizants. There is no fat and the gland was quite dense so his gynecomastia was treated through the areola. Postoperative views (below) at 12 months.

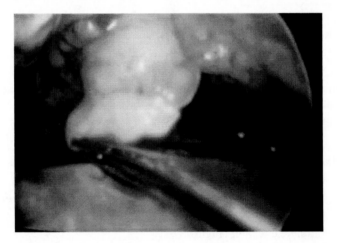

Figure 8. Transaxillary endoscopic view of the subareolar gland.

We think one of the critical points in surgery of the gynecomastia is to know how much gland has to be left under the areola to avoid its collapse and retraction. If too much, the areola will be pulled by the pectoralis muscle. If too little, the patient will complain that he still has gynecomastia. Our approach is to leave the same thickness as the surrounding skin, to leave the most homogeneous flap on the chest. The compressive girdle and massaging will help the flap to adapt over the muscle.

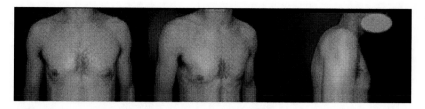

Figure 9. A 28-year-old male patient with type I gynecomastia treated through the axilla. Postoperative view at 10 months.

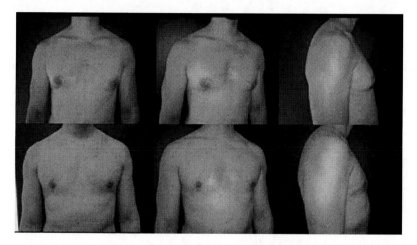

Figure 10. Grade I/II gynecomastia in a 24-year-old male patient with mastectomy performed through the axilla. Postoperative view at 12 months.

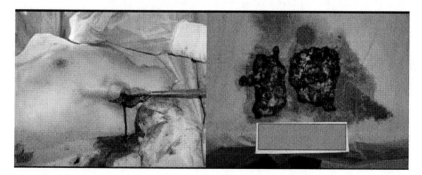

Figure 11. Operative view with the specimen retrieved through the axilla (left) and the excised tissue from both sides (right).

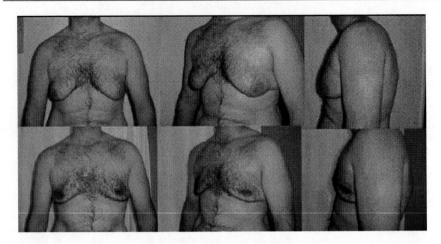

Figure 12. A 49-year-old male patient with grade IV gynecomastia and ptosis type III. We performed tissue reduction with the de Prado's technique. One year after the treatment we can observe the good shrinkage achieved although there is some skin excess. The patient refused to have further treatments.

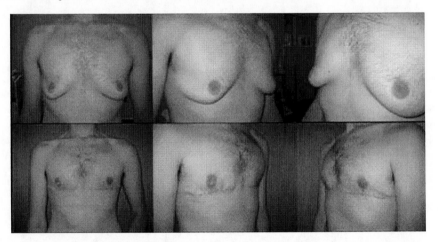

Figure 13. A 17-year-old male patient with grade IV gynecomastia and breast ptosis. The chosen technique in this case was mastectomy with horizontal skin excision. Postoperative view at 12 months.

We propose the following algorithm for the surgical treatment of gynecomastia (Figure 17) [45, 46]:

- Grade I (mainly glandular): Areolar or axillary excision of the gland
- Grade II: Liposuction plus shaver; in cases with a strong glandular component, consider an areolar or axillary approach to remove the gland
- Grade III: Liposuction plus shaver
- Grade IV: First-stage treatment with liposuction plus shaver to reduce volume; consider skin removal 1 year post treatment, if needed.

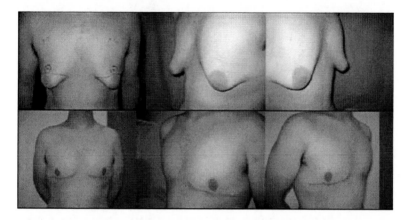

Figure 14. An 18-year-old male patient with grade IV gynecomastia and breast with a tuberous-like shape. A horizontal mastectomy and elevation of the nipple areola complex were performed. Postoperative views at 8 months.

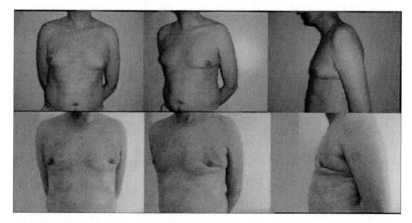

Figure 15. Dimpling and skin retraction after de Prado's technique in a 45-year-old patient with grade III gynecomastia.

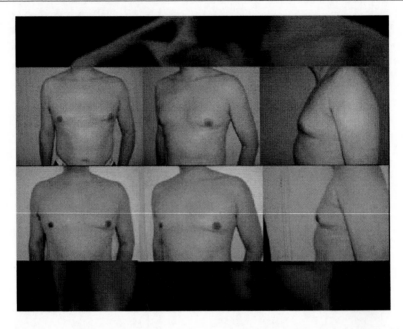

Figure 16. Insufficient resection at the left side of this 36-year-old male patient with type II gynecomastia.

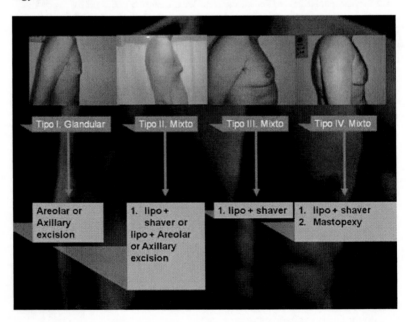

Figure 17. Our algorithm for surgical treatment of gynecomastia.

References

[1] Chavoushi S. H., Ghabili K., Kazemi, A., Aslanabadi, A., Babapour S., Ahmedii R., Golzari S. E. J. *Surgery for Gynecomastia in the Islamic Golden Age:* Al-Tasrif of Al-Zahrawi (936-1013 AD). ISRN Surgery, Volume 2012, 5 pages.

[2] Barros A. C., Sampaio M. C. Ginecomastia: Fisiopatologia, avaliação e tratamento. *Sao Paulo Med J.* 2012; 130:187-97.

[3] Carlson H. E. Approach to the patient with gynecomastia. *J Clin Endocrinol Metab.* 2011; 96:15-21.

[4] Bembo S. A., Carlson H. E. Gynecomastia: Its features, and when and how to treat it. *Cleve Clin J Med.* 2004; 71:511-7.

[5] Cordova A., Moschella F. Algorithm for clinical evaluation and surgical treatment of gynaecomastia. *J Plast Reconstr Aesthet Surg.* 2008; 61:41-9.

[6] Ratnam B. V. A new classification and treatment protocol for gynecomastia. *Aesthet Surg J.* 2009; 29:26-31.

[7] Simon B. E., Hoffman S., Kahn S. Classification and surgical correction of gynecomastia. *Plast Reconstr Surg.* 1973; 27:48-52.

[8] Rohrich R. J., Ha R. Y., Kenkel J. M. et al. Classification and management of gynaecomastia: defining the role of ultrasound-assisted liposuction. *Plast Reconstr Surg* 2003; 111:909-23.

[9] Williams M. J. Gynecomastia: its incidence, recognition and host characterization in 447 autopsy cases. *Am J Med.* 1963; 34:103-12.

[10] Bannayan G. A., Hajdu S. I. Gynecomastia: clinicopathologic study of 351 cases. *Am J Clin Pathol.* 1972; 57: 431-437.

[11] Andersen J. A., Gram J. B. Gynecomasty: histological aspects in a surgical material. *Acta Pathol Microbiol Immunol Scand.* 1982; 90A: 185-90.

[12] Nicolis G. L., Modlinger R. S., Gabrilove J. L. A study of the histopathology of human gynecomastia. *J Clin Endocrinol Metab.* 1971; 32:173-8.

[13] Johnson R. E., Murad M. H. Gynecomastia: Pathophysiology, Evaluation, and Management Concise Review for Clinicians. *Mayo Clin Proc.* 2009; 84:1010-1015.

[14] Granick C. J. S., Granick M. S. Gynecomastia. What the surgeon needs to know. *Open Access Journal of Plastic Surgery,* 2009, Jan 15, 41-51.

[15] Mahoney C. P. Adolescent gynecomastia differential diagnosis and management. *Pediatr Clin N Am.* 1990; 37:1389-404.

[16] Draghi F., Tarantino C. C., Madonia L., Ferrozzi G. Ultrasonography of the male breast. *J Ultrasound* (2011) 14, 122e-129.

[17] Niewoehner C. B., Anna E., Schorer A. E., Catherine B. Gynaecomastia and breast cancer in men. *BMJ* 2008; 336:709-13.

[18] Frazier A. A. *Three patterns of male gynecomastia.* Radiographics.rsna. org. March-April 2013, page 460.

[19] Parker L. N., Gray D. R., Lai M. K., Levin E. R. Treatment of gynecomastia with tamoxifen: A double blind crossover study. *Metabolism,* 1986, 35:705-708.

[20] Lawrence S. E., Faught K. A., Vethamuthu J., Lawson M. L. Beneficial effects of raloxifene and tamoxifen in the treatment of pubertal gynecomastia. *J Pediatr.* 2004; 145:71-6.

[21] Derman O., Kanbur N. O., Kutluk T. Tamoxifen treatment for pubertal gynecomastia. *Int J Adolesc Med Health.* 2003; 15:359-63.

[22] Khan H. N., Rampaul R., Blamey R. W. Management of physiological gynecomastia with tamoxifen. *Breast,* 2004, 13:61-65.

[23] Hanavadi S., Banerjee D., Monypenny I. J., Mansel R. E. The role of tamoxifen in the management of gynecomastia. *Breast* 2006, 15: 276-280.

[24] Devoto C. Enzo, Madariaga A. Marcia, Lioi C. Ximena, Mardones Nelly. Influence of size and duration of gynecomastia on its response to treatment with tamoxifen. *Rev. Méd. Chile* 2007; 135: 1558-1565.

[25] Riepe F. G. 1., Baus I., Wiest S., Krone N., Sippell W. G., Partsch C. J. Treatment of pubertal gynecomastia with the specific aromatase inhibitor anastrozole. *Horm Res.* 2004; 62(3):113-8. Epub 2004 Jul 20.

[26] Fruhstorfer B. H., Malata C. M. A systematic approach to the surgical treatment of gynaecomastia. *Br J Plast Surg.* 2003; 27:237-246.

[27] Webster J. P. Mastectomy for gynecomastia through a semicircular intra-areolar incision. *Ann Surg.* 1946; 27:557-575.

[28] Kinsella C., Landfair A., Rottgers S. A. et al. The Psychological Burden of Idiopathic Adolescent Gynecomastia. *Plast. Reconstr. Surg,* 2012, 129:1-7.

[29] Nuzzi J., Cerrato F. E., Erikson C. R. et al. Psychosocial Impact of Adolescent Gynecomastia: A Prospective Case-Control Study. *Plast. Reconstr. Surg,* 2013, 131: 890-896.

[30] Crerand C. E., Magee L. Cosmetic and Reconstructive Breast Surgery in adolescents: Psychological, ethical, and Legal Considerations. *Semin Plast Surg* 2013; 27:72-78.

[31] Illouz Y.-G. Body contouring by lipolysis: A 5-year experience with over 3000 cases. *Plast Reconstr Surg* 1983; 72:591-7.

[32] Zocchi M. Ultrasonic liposculpturing. *Aesthetic Plast Surg* 1992; 16:287-98.

[33] Hodgson E. L., Fruhstorfer B. H., Malata C. M. Ultrasonic liposuction in the treatment of gynecomastia. *Plast Reconstr Surg* 2005; 116:646-653.

[34] Rohrich R. J., Beran S. J., Fodor P. B. The role of subcutaneous infiltration in suction-assisted lipoplasty: A review. *Plast Reconstr Surg* 1997; 99:514-519.

[35] Trelles M. A., Mordon S. R., Bonanad E. et al. Laser-assisted lipolysis in the treatment of gynecomastia: A prospective study in 28 patients. *Laser Med Sci.* 2013; 28:375-382.

[36] Trelles, M. A., Alcolea, J. M., Bonanad, E., Moreno-Moraga, J., Leclère, F. M. Liposucción láser-asistida en ginecomastia: Seguimiento ecográfico y estadístico de los efectos observados de retracción cutánea. *Cir. plást. iberolatinoam.* 2013, 39: 121-127.

[37] Morselli P. G. "Pull-through": A new technique for breast reduction in gynecomastia. *Plast Reconstr Surg,* 1996, 97:450-454.

[38] Morselli P. G., Morellini A. Breast reshaping in gynecomastia by the "pull-through technique": Considerations after 15 years. *Eur J Plast Surg* 2012; 35:365-371.

[39] Blugerman G., Schalvezon D., Mulholland R. S., Soto J. A., Siguen M. Gynecomastia treatment using radio frequency-assisted liposuction. *Eur J Plast Surg,* 2013, 36:231-236.

[40] Hamas R. S., Williams Ch. W. A Sharp Cutting Liposuction Cannula for Gynecomastia. *Aesth. Surg. J.*1998; 18: 261-265.

[41] Prado A. C., Castillo P. F. Minimal surgical access to treat gynecomastia with the use of a power-assisted arthroscopic-endoscopic cartilage shaver. *Plast Reconstr Surg* 2005; 115:939-942.

[42] Haddad Filho D., Garcia Arruda R., Alonso N. Treatment of Severe Gynecomastia (Grade III) by Resection of Periareolar Skin. *Aesthetic Surgery Journal* 2006 26: 669-673.

[43] Persichetti P., Berloco M., Casadei R. M. et al. Gynecomastia and the Complete Circumareolar Approach in the Surgical Management of Skin Redundancy. *Plast Reconstr Surg,* 2001, 107:948-954.

[44] Gheita A. Gynecomastia: The Horizontal Ellipse Method for Its Correction. *Aesth Plast Surg* 2008, 32:795-801.

[45] Benito-Ruiz J., Raigosa M., Manzano M., Salvador L. Assessment of a suction-assisted cartilage shaver plus liposuction for the treatment of gynecomastia. *Aesthet Surg J.* 2009; 29:302-309.

[46] Benito-Ruiz J., Raigosa M., Manzano M., Salvador L. Nuevo paradigma del tratamiento quirúrgico de la ginecomastia. *Cir. Plást. iberolatinoam.* 2013, 39:121-127.

[47] Lapid, O., & Jolink, F. Surgical management of gynecomastia: 20 years' experience. *Scandinavian Journal of Surgery,* 2014, 103(1), 41-45.

In: Endocrine Diseases
Editor: Kenneth Hines

ISBN: 978-1-63482-592-4
© 2015 Nova Science Publishers, Inc.

Chapter 2

Etiopathogenesis and Genetics of Gynecomastia

Michael Stamatakos[1,], Konstantinos Ntzeros[2]*
and Konstantinos Kontzoglou[3]
[1]Nursing Unit of Molaoi, General Hospital of Lakonia, Molaoi, Greece
[2]Astros Medical Center, Panarcadian General Hospital of Tripoli,
Tripoli, Greece
[3]2nd Department of Propaedeutic Surgery, Medical School,
University of Athens, Laiko General Hospital,
Athens, Greece

Abstract

Gynecomastia is a benign disease defined by enlargement of the male mammary gland. Dysregulation of the androgen-estrogen balance is the main underlying mechanism. The most common form of this disease is the physiologic gynecomastia, caused by normal transient or permanent changes. It is characterized by three peaks of prevalence at the neonatal, pubertal, and adult period. The neonatal gynecomastia is transient and resolves within a year, while the underlying cause is the maternal-placental estrogens, which circulate in the neonate. The pubertal

* E-mail: mixalislak@gmail.com.

gynecomastia is transient and resolves within two years. The underlying cause is an estrogen increase due to testicular stimulation by gonadotrophins. The adult gynecomastia is observed mainly in men aged 50 to 80 years and it is correlated with physiologic changes of aged-related change, such as a decline in androgen levels, increase of adipose tissue and increased aromatase activity resulting in an upregulation of circulating estrogens. However, except from the physiologic causes of gynecomastia there are also pathologic ones covering a wide range of different diseases. The pathologic gynecomastia affects men in any age and does not follow the three peaks pattern of prevalence observed at the physiologic form. The pathologic reasons can be divided into three categories: a) systemic diseases comprising tumors producing hormones and chronic diseases of liver and kidneys. b) Endocrinological diseases including thyroid, adrenal, gonadal, and pituitary dysfunction. c) Iatrogenic causes and exogenous agents, which develop into gynecomastia through different mechanisms, such as direct action of estrogens or estrogen-like substances and inhibition of androgen production or androgen receptor's function.

These agents are pharmaceutical substances used for diseases such as hypertension, congestive heart failure, HIV infection, gastroesophageal reflux disease, benign prostate hyperplasia and prostate cancer. Gynecomastia has a strong genetic background. It is developed in several disorders of sexual hormones or organs derived from chromosomal anomalies, gene mutations, and polymorphisms. Common syndromes such as Klinefelter's and Peutz-Jeghers as well as rare syndromes such as Borjeson-Forssman-Lehmann are described to have gynecomastia as one of the characteristic anomalies. Other disorders related to gynecomastia are the aromatase excess syndrome, Kennedy's disease, and androgen insensitivity syndrome. Finally, there are polymorphisms in genes such as *CYP19*, *ERS2*, and *LEPR*, which are shown to be the causative factor of gynectomastia.

Gynecomastia is considered a benign disorder without a strong correlation with breast cancer, except in the case of Klinefelter's syndrome. The cause of pathologic gynecomastia could vary from the administration of an exogenous agent to the polymorphism of a single gene. Therefore, males should be examined and investigated for a causative factor with great attention especially when gynecomastia is accompanied with infertility.

Introduction

Definitions

Gynecomastia is a benign, abnormal enlargement of the male breast gland, which results from proliferation of the glandular, fibrous, and adipose components of the breast. It is the most common breast condition in men. The main underlying cause is an increased estrogen action due to the imbalance of free estrogen and androgen activity or an increased estrogen-to-androgen ratio. The overall prevalence is estimated to range within 30 to 50% but there is a specific trimodal age distribution (Karnath, 2008). The first peak of prevalence is observed at infancy or the neonatal period, the second peak during puberty, and the last peak in older males aged from 50 to 80 years. This distribution pattern is usually connected with asymptomatic gynecomastia and it is classified as the physiologic type of this benign disease. The neonatal gynecomastia is transient and resolves within a year, with the underlying cause being the maternal-placental estrogens, which circulate in the neonate. The pubertal gynecomastia is transient and resolves within two years. The underlying cause is an estrogen increase due to testicular stimulation by gonadotrophins. The adult gynecomastia is observed mainly in men aged 50 to 80 years and it is correlated with physiologic changes of aged-related hypogonadism, such as a decline in androgen levels, increase of adipose tissue and aromatase activity resulting in upregulation of circulating estrogens. The development of gynecomastia from a number of medical conditions, medication drugs, or exogenous substances is classified as pathologic gynecomastia. There is not any specific distribution age pattern. The pathologic reasons can be divided into three categories: a) systemic diseases comprising tumors producing estradiol or hCG and chronic diseases such as hepatic cirrhosis and chronic kidney disease. b) Endocrinological diseases including thyroid, adrenal, gonadal, and pituitary dysfunction. c) Iatrogenic causes and exogenous agents, which develop gynecomastia through different mechanisms, such as direct action of estrogens or estrogen-like substances and inhibition of androgen production or androgen receptor's function. Finally, there is the idiopathic gynecomastia, which is of unknown etiopathologic reasons and it is the most commonly diagnosed type. It constitutes 25% of all the diagnosed cases. Several hypotheses have been proposed to explain the development of gynecomastia in patients with normal concentrations of pituitary and sex hormones as well as sex-hormone-binding-globulin (SHBG; Ismail and Barth, 2001).

Physiology of Male Mammary Gland

A. Mammary Development

The fetal development of the human breast can be divided into two periods. The first comprises the development of the primary mammary bud, which takes place into the first trimester, and the second period comprises the development of a primary mammary gland, expanding at the rest of the intrauterine life (Javed and Lteif, 2013). It is important to mention that the early stages of breast development (mainly during the first trimester) do not depend on hormonal stimuli, while during the second trimester hormones have a crucial role in this developmental process (Robinson et al., 1999; Turashvili et al., 2005). However, no differentiation between the two sexes is observed during the fetal period.

The first signs of breast development are observed during the 4th to 7th week of gestation with the existence and proliferation of progenitor cells at the superficial layer of two thoracic regions. Subsequently, the mammary crests or milk lines are formed. Later the mammary crests regress, remaining only the two primary mammary buds at the pectoral region (Javed and Lteif, 2013). Nearing the end of the first trimester, the primary mammary buds infiltrate the underlying mesenchyme and increase in size. Additionally, this infiltration stimulates the surrounding mesenchyme to differentiate to fibroblast-like cells, creating a zone of supporting cells (Jolicoeur, 2005). At the end of the first trimester, the infiltration of the upper dermis has been completed and the supporting zone contains fibroblasts, smooth muscle cells, capillary endothelial cells, and adypocytes (Javedand Lteif, 2013).

At the second trimester the mammary bud develops transversely as well as vertically, forming the secondary epithelial bud, which elongates vertically surrounding the primary mammary bud (Javedand Lteif, 2013). Subsequently, the secondary buds canalize and merge forming the lactiferous ducts. The outer layer of the lactiferous ducts differentiates to myoepithelial cells while the inner layer differentiates to secretory cells (Jolicoeur, 2005). At the end of the second trimester the fundamental structure of the mammary gland is completed.

During the third trimester, the secondary epithelial buds continue to increase in size with new branches and the lactiferous canal system elongates (Jolicoeur, 2005). The supporting fibroconnective layer of the mammary gland increases in vascularity and the circulating hormones of the fetus, produced by the maternal-placental interface, might induce a secretory activity of the mammary gland (Jolicoeur, 2005). However, there is disagreement over whether the mammary gland at the end of the third trimester contains only ductal structures or lobural as well (Javedand Lteif, 2013). It is estimated that 15 to 20 lobes of the mammary gland are formed during pregnancy. Additionally, during the third trimester other structures of the human breast develop such as the nipple, the surrounding areola, and the supportive ligaments (Javedand Lteif, 2013).

The postnatal period of breast development is confined within the first two years; afterwards the normal mammary gland remains inactive until puberty. At birth, there is no difference between the male and female infant as far as the presentation of the breast is concerned (Jayasingheet al., 2010).

During the first few months after birth, there is a progressive transition from the maternal-placental hormones to the infant's gonadal hormones. During the fall of the maternal-placental hormones, the infant prolactin increases resulting in breast enlargement and in some cases secretion of milk (Anbazhaganet al., 1991).

Another important issue is the development of nipples' erectile mechanism and the pigmentation of areolae, which are observed to take place in the very early period after birth.

Subsequently, other morphological and functional changes of the mammary gland occur but finally this process regresses into small ductal structures surrounded by fibroblastic stroma at the end of the second year (Javedand Lteif, 2013).

During puberty, no further development of the male mammary gland is observed, except from the cases of gynecomastia where there is secondary ductal and stromal but not lobular hypertrophy (Howard and Gusterson, 2000). The only change in the male breast during puberty is an increase in nipple diameter.

As for the female breast, it undergoes numerous anatomical and histological changes. The most important anatomical changes are described by the Tanner scale, describing the five stages of development (Table 1).

The histological changes start with an increase in fibroconnective and adipose tissue of the stroma, which precedes the ductal enlongation and dichotomous branching of the ductal structures. As for the lobular structures, they develop mainly up to the lobule type 1 while the rest of the types require further maturation processes available during pregnancy and lactation. The main stimuli for breast development during puberty are the estrogen surge for the females, while the major inhibiting factor for breast development in males is the testosterone surge.

However, even in females the estrogen surge is not enough to initiate and complete the developmental changes required for fulfilling this process. Other hormones such as the pituitary growth hormone and some important growth factors are required.

Table 1. Major anatomical changes in female breast described by the Tanner scale

Stage 1	Elevation of the papilla
Stage 2	Formation of breast bud, elevation of the nipple and the surrounding tissues and increase in areola's diameter
Stage 3	Further enlargement of the breast and the areola, increase in nipple diameter
Stage4	Further enlargement of the breast and elevation, areola and nipple forming a secondary mound projecting from the contour of the surrounding breast, increase in nipple diameter
Stage 5	Breast reaching its adult size, the areola recess to general contour of the surrounding breast but the papilla is still projecting, increase in nipple diameter

B. Effect of Sex Hormones in Male Breast

a. Origin of Sex Hormones in Males

Sex hormones in males are produced in three regions: the testes, adrenal glands, and extraglandular sites. In the testes 95% of circulating testosterone is produced as well as a small fraction of circulating estrogens (15% of estradiol and 5% estrone; Barros and Sampaio, 2012). The rest of androgens are produced in adrenal glands with androstenedione being the major androgen. However, the remainder of estrogen in males is produced in extraglandular sites through the process of androgen aromatization. The major aromatization sites in males are intramammary and subcutaneous fat (Barros and Sampaio, 2012). Other sites are liver, skin, muscles, and kidneys. Cytochrome P450 aromatase converts testosterone to estradiol and androstenedione to estrone.

b. Effect of Estrogens and Androgens in the Male Breast

In general, estrogens stimulate and androgens inhibit breast development both in males and females. Estrogens are shown to induce ductal epithelial tissue proliferation resulting in ductal elongation and branching. Additionally, they induce proliferation of the ductal supportive tissues and vessels. On the other hand, progesterone, which males normally lack, induces side-branching and secretory alveolar development. Androgens are shown to inhibit breast development in many cases, such as in women with androgen excess where they suppress breast development even when there are adequate concentrations of circulating estrogens (Dimitrakakis and Bondy, 2009).

Etiopathogenesis

Physiologic Gynecomastia

A. Neonatal Gynecomastia

Neonatal gynecomastia is defined as the presence of a palpable mammary gland behind the areolas in newborns, even if such breast enlargement might not be identified by vision. It is a common benign condition affecting 60 to 90% of newborns (Derkacz et al., 2011). Both of the mammary glands are usually affected and galactorhea might be observed in up to 5% of neonates (Karnath, 2008). Neonatal gynecomastia is a benign transient condition, which resolves within a few months up to the first year.

The underlying cause of this condition is the maternal-placental estrogens that are transferred to the fetus and stimulate the fetal mammary glands to develop further. The breast gland development is enhanced during the third trimester of pregnancy by the maternal-placental hormones, which are transferred to the fetus and continue to exert their action during the early postnatal period. However, there is a strong hypothesis about the role of endogenous mammotrophic hormones, which could contribute to neonatal breast development (Schmidt et al., 2002). It is also shown that during the early postnatal period, the infant's endocrine system secretes considerable reproductive hormones (Andersson et al., 1998). Therefore, the gynecomastia at the neonatal period might be a more complicated condition with synergistic action of both maternal-placental and infant's hormones.

Another important issue is the accompanying galactorhea in newborns with gynecomastia. Neonatal milk is also known as "witch's milk" in some folklore stories (Karnath, 2008). It is well known that prolactin is a hormone that promotes milk secretion and its increase coincides with the decrease of progesterone concentration (McKiernan and Hull, 1981). Additionally, prolactin is a hormone that it is not transferred through the placenta. Therefore, the newborn's galactorhea is attributed to an endogenous prolactin surge following a decrease of the circulating neonatal progesterone (McKiernan and Hull, 1981). Fetal prolactin during the third trimester of pregnancy is increased while it declines within the first weeks after delivery in full term newborns (McKiernan and Hull, 1981).

B. Pubertal Gynecomastia

Pubertal gynecomastia affects 20-70% of young males and the peak age of developing gynecomastia is 13 to 14 years (Derkacz et al., 2011). It is usually transient and moderate and it regresses within 2 years. The underlying cause is the deregulation of the estrogen to androgen ratio during the stimulation of the testes from gonadotropins. During puberty, testosterone levels increase 30-fold but estradiol levels also increase 3-fold. However, the estradiol increase precedes the testosterone one, resulting in a deregulation of the androgen to estrogen ratio. This estrogen increase contributes to the extraglandular aromatization of the testicular and adrenal androgens. Additionally, there is a genetic study which indicates that except for the increased estrogen level, gynecomastia might be associated with specific polymorphisms of estrogen receptor beta, supporting the genetic background of this benign condition (Eren et al., 2014).

Leptin is another important player in pubertal gynecomastia since it is associated with increased aromatase activity in adipose cells and breast tissues (Dundar et al., 2005). Additionally, it is believed to have a direct effect in stimulating the growth of breast cells. The presence of increased leptin levels in males with pubertal gynecomastia and the identification of a specific leptin receptor's polymorphism that affects susceptibility to gynecomastia, indicates the possible direct or indirect role of leptin in this benign condition (Eren et al., 2014; Dundar et al., 2005).

C. Scenescent Gynecomastia

The third peak of prevalence in physiologic gynecomastia is observed in men 50 to 80 years of age. This kind of gynecomastia is supported by three natural consequences of the aging process. Firstly, it is the hypogonadism, which results in a decrease of testosterone production and an increase of sex hormone binding globulin (SHBG; Leifke et al., 2000). Both of these events result in diminishing the free testosterone plasma levels. Secondly, it is the accumulation of adipose tissue, which contributes to the extraglandular estrogen production through aromatase activity. Thirdly, there are men who have increased luteinizing hormone (LH) levels during senescence. Chronic LH stimulation of the testis would result in increased secretion of testicular estrogen (Ismail and Barth, 2001). The decreased testosterone production and the estrogen elevated levels during senescence results in disruption of the estrogen-to-androgen balance, which in turn enables the development of gynecomastia.

Pathologic Gynecomastia

Pathologic gynecomastia comprises several cases where there is an underlying pathophysiological process triggering mammary gland development and it is usually accompanied with other symptoms. The causes of pathologic gynecomastia can be classified using several criteria but two proposed ways are described.

The first way is using the underlying pathologic process, which causes gynecomastia, as major classifying criterion. Three categories are created: a) Systemic diseases comprising tumors and chronic diseases. b) Endocrinological diseases including thyroid, adrenal, gonadal, and pituitary dysfunction. c) Exogenous or acquired causes, which develop gynecomastia through different mechanisms. The second approach of classification is based on the levels and balance of sex hormones. There are four major categories: a) Estrogen Excess, b) Androgen deficiency, c) Altered estrogen to androgen balance, d) Decreased androgen action. Table 2 shows the main hormonal disturbances observed in some well-known diseases associated with gynecomastia. In this manuscript, the first way of classifying the pathologic processes associated with gynecomastia is used.

Table 2. Hormonal disturbances in gynecomastia-related diseases

Underlying disease	Estrogens	Testicular Androgens	PRL	FSH	LH	SHBG	Thyroid hormones	Adrenal androgens	E/A ratio
Chronic kidney failure	↑	↓	↗	–	↑	–	–	–	↑
Dialysis	↑ due to lag in liver function	–	–	N	N	–	–	–	↑
Liver Diseases	↑	↓	N or ↗	–	–	↑	N or decreased response to TRH	↑	↑
Hyperthyroidism	↑ levels of free estradiol	↓ levels of free testosterone	–	–	–	↑	↑ levels of thyroid hormones	↑	↑
Malnourishment-Refeeding Gynecomastia	↑ due to lag in liver function	–	–	N	N	–	–	–	↑
Primary Hypogonadism	↑	↓	–	↑	↑	–	–	–	↑
Secondary Hypogonadism	N	↓	–	↓	↓	–	–	–	↑
B-HCG producing Tumors	↑	N or ↓	–	↓	↓	–	–	–	↑
Feminizing Adrenal Tumors	↑	↓	–	↓	↓	–	–	↑	↑
Prolactinomas	↑	↓	↑	–	↓	–	–	–	↑

↑: Increase, ↓: Decrease, N: Normal, ↗: Slightly Increased, –: Not Referred.

A. Systemic Diseases

Malnourishment-Refeeding Gynecomastia

Gynecomastia developed in malnourished persons after returning to a normal diet. It was first observed after the end of World War II (Derkacz et al., 2011).

The mechanism of this procedure is based on two sequential events. Firstly, the malnourishment resulting in severe weight loss is associated with secondary hypogonadism due to decreased gonadotropin production. The established hypogonadism results in decreased testosterone secretion while the estrogen levels remain at normal values due to physiological production by peripheral conversion of adrenal androgens (Cuhaci et al., 2014). The second event is the refeeding process, which results in increased production of the gonadotropins, testosterone and estradiol. However, there is a decreased metabolism rate of estrogen due to the liver recovery lag, resulting in a transiently increased estrogen to androgen ratio, which promotes the development of gynecomastia (Dickson, 2012).

Gynecomastia regresses within two years without any intervention. This situation is also named as "second puberty" and it is also observed in chronic kidney failure patients entering dialysis.

Chronic Kidney Failure and Dialysis

Gynecomastia is quite a common symptom of patients with chronic renal disease and it is observed in 18 to 50% of patients undergoing dialysis (Zamd et al., 2004; Cuhaci et al., 2014). However, there are differences between the patients undergoing dialysis and those who are not, as long as the causative factor of developing gynecomastia is concerned. The underlying reasons in patients with chronic kidney failure are some hormonal disturbances, which change the estrogens-to-androgens ratio in favor of estrogens. More specifically, there is a decrease in serum testosterone, an increase in estrogen and LH serum levels, and a small increase in serum prolactin (PRL; Derkacz et al., 2011). On the other hand, gynecomastia of dialysispatients is attributed to the malnourishment-refeeding mechanism. Patients with kidney failure prior to dialysis are usually at low BMI and malnourished due to the strict diet that they are supposed to follow as part of their disease management. When they start dialysis courses, the diet restrictions are diminished and they usually gain weight. Malnutrition affects the hypothalamic-pituitary-gonadal axis diminishing the secretion of gonadotrophins and decreasing the production of testicular testosterone because of hypogonadism (Cuhaci et al., 2014).

However, when the patient starts to gain weight, pituitary and gonadal hormones are produced at normal rates but there is a liver lag in recovery, which results in lower levels of estrogen degradation (Dickson, 2012). This means that for a short period the estrogens to androgens balance is disrupted in favor of estrogen, triggering the development of gynecomastia. Therefore, this kind of gynecomastia is transient and resolves after one or two years. On the other hand, gynecomastia of patients developed from hormonal disturbances during the course of chronic renal failure is not affected by dialysis and resolves only when kidney transplantation is successful (Derkacz et al., 2011).

Liver Diseases

The main pathophysiologic process of liver diseases resulting in gynecomastia is based on increased levels of circulating estrogens and decreased free testosterone. Firstly, the dysfunction of the liver itself results in decreased hepatic degradation of estrogens and increased production of SHBG (Dickson, 2012). Subsequently, there is increased production of adrenal androgens and decreased degradation of the liver, resulting in increased circulating levels of these androgens, which are aromatized peripherally to estrogens, enhancing the estrogen excess (Cuhaci et al., 2014). Finally, there is a down-regulation of androgen receptors in patients with liver disease (Karnath, 2008).

Gynecomastia is observed in 40 to 60% of patients with cirrhosis of the liver (Karnath, 2008). Alcohol-induced cirrhosis is often associated with secondary hypogonadism due to disruption of the hypothalamic-pituitary-testicular axis, resulting in decreased testosterone production (Derkacz et al., 2011; Cuhaci et al., 2014). Additionally, in alcohol-induced cirrhosis some patients have increased prolactin levels and a decreased response to TRH (Derkacz et al., 2011). On the other hand, in non-alcohol-induced cirrhosis, patients had increased levels of circulating progesterone, which is not observed in alcohol-related cirrhotic patients (Derkacz et al., 2011). Progesterone is a stimulatory factor of breast development. Finally, there are liver malignancies, which can promote gynecomastia either due to increased production of estrogen from the tumor itself (malignant hepatoma) or increased aromatase activity in the tumor (Derkacz et al., 2011; Cuhaci et al., 2014).

Tumor Associated Gynecomastia

Gynecomastia is related with four main categories of tumors: a) the β-HCG producing tumors, b) the feminizing adrenal tumors, c) the testicular tumors, and d) the pituitary adenomas, which produce prolactin (prolactinomas).

- β-HCG producing tumors:
  Normally, males have undetectable levels of β-HCG. However, the development of some tumors results in high levels of secreted β-HCG. β-HCGproducing tumors account for 3% of all cases of gynecomastia(Ismail and Barth, 2001). Some of them have also the ability to convert adrenal androgens to estrogens through the aromatization process. They are divided into two main categories, the testicular germ cell tumors such as choriocarcinoma, and the tumors of ectopic origin such as large-cell lung, gastric, renal cell carcinomas, and hepatoma or hepatoblastoma (mainly in pre-adolescent males; Cuhaci et al., 2014; Dickson, 2012).
  The underlying mechanism of developing gynecomastia in such tumors is associated with the structural resemblance between β-HCGand LH. β-HCG stimulates Leydig cells to initiate testicular steroidogenesis and more specifically, the production of estradiol (Barros and Sampaio, 2012). The estradiol levels increase 4-7 times while testosterone remains at normal levels (Ismail and Barth, 2001). Subsequently, the testicular produced estradiol has a negative feedback on gonadotropin production and it also suppresses the androgen production in testes (Ismail and Barth, 2001). Finally, the β-HCG continuous stimulation downregulated the β-HCG/ LH receptors in testis, which in turn decrease the testicular steroidogenesis while the serum estrogens remain at elevated levels (Ismail and Barth, 2001). This disrupted estrogen-to-androgen ratio enables the development of gynecomastia.
- Feminizing adrenal tumors:
  Another important category of tumors associated with gynecomastia are the adrenal ones, which secrete estrogen or have a mixed secretion of estrogen and androgen precursors such as androstenedione or DHEA. They are also named as feminizing adrenal tumors due to the obvious effects of produced estrogens to the secondary sex characteristics. Except for gynecomastia, other clinical symptoms are breast tenderness, gonadal deficiency, with or without lowered libido, and ejaculation problems (Chentliet al., 2013). Such tumors account for 0.37 to 2% of all adrenal tumors (Chentliet al., 2013). They usually are large and are usually malignant even though they might

seem benign (Barros and Sampaio, 2012). Feminizing adrenal tumors more frequently observed in older men, 70+, years old (7%), than in younger men, aged less than 30 years (1%), and more rarely in women and children (Chentliet al., 2013). The pathogenetic mechanism is quite simple since the increased estrogen levels downregulate gonadotropin production, which in turn results in decreased testosterone production (Barros and Sampaio, 2012). The detection of such cases is based on the increased serum DHEA-sulfate and urinary 17-ketosteroids levels (Dickson, 2012).

- Testicular tumors:
  Testicular cancer is one of the most common malignancies observed in young males. About 10% of testicular cancers develop gynecomastia before the presence of a palpable testicular lump. The main categoriesof testicular tumors associated with gynecomastia are Leydig and Sertoli cell tumors, known to secrete estrogens (Barros and Sampaio, 2012). In Leydig cell tumors the presence of symptoms related to increased estrogen production might be observed in up to 20% of cases (Derkacz et aI., 2011). Leydig cell tumors can occur at any age, but they are mostly observed in young boys (5 to 10 years old) and men (aged 25 to 35 years). Most of Sertoli and Leydig cell tumors are benign. The main underlying mechanism of developing gynecomastia in these estrogen-producing tumors is based on the negative feedback of high estrogen levels on LH production. The decrease of LH levels downregulates testicular steroidogenesis while the increased estrogen levels stimulate SHBG synthesis (Derkacz et al., 2011). The combination of these events results in increased levels of free estradiol and low levels of free testosterone, supporting the development of mammary gland.

- Prolactinomas:
  Pituitary adenomas producing prolactin are one of the main reasons causing hypeprolactinaemia resulting in nipple discharge and gynecomastia in male patients. However, not all patients with hyperprolactinaemia develop gynecomastia. The pathogenetic mechanism of gynecomastia in these patients is based on the inhibitory effect of prolactin on LH secretion. Low levels of LH lead to decreased production of testosterone and increased production of estrogen from Leydig cells.

B. Endocrinological Diseases

Thyroid Dysfunction

Thyroid dysfunction and especially hyperthyroidism is associated with gynecomastia from 10 to 40% while hypothyroidism is rarely associated with this benign disease. The main underlying mechanism in hyperthyroidism is the increased liver production of SHBG and the enhanced adrenal production of steroids (Derkacz et al., 2011). Additionally, there is increased peripheral conversion of androgen to estrogen. High levels of SHBG result in low levels of free testosterone and increased levels of free estradiol. The increased production of adrenal androgens, in accordance with the enhanced peripheral aromatization process, establishes the estrogen excess. The underlying mechanism of gynecomastia in hypothyroidism is not fully understood. However, it is supported that there are low levels of testosterone, which in turn stimulate LH production, increasing estradiol levels (Karnath, 2008).

Hypogonadism Related Gynecomastia

Male hypogonadism results from failure of the testis to produce normal levels of testosterone and normal numbers of spermatozoa (Dandona and Rosenberg, 2010). It is divided into primary hypogonadism where there is a gonadal dysfunction and secondary hypogonadism where there is a dysfunction of the hypothalamic-pituitary axis. In primary hypogonadism the testes fail to produce normal amounts of testosterone while there are high levels of LH and FSH concentrations and it is also named as hypergonadotropic hypogonadism. In secondary hypogonadism, the problem is located on the hypothalamus-pituitary axis while the testis has normal functionality. However, due to low levels of FSH and LH resulting in subnormal stimulation of testes, there is low testosterone production (Dandona and Rosenberg, 2010). This kind of hypogonadism is also named hypogonadotropic hypogonadism. Table 3 shows different causes of primary and secondary hypogonadism.

The underlying mechanism of gynecomastia in patients with primary hypogonadism is associated firstly with the low serum levels of testosterone resulting from the gonadal dysfunction. Secondly, there are increased serum levels of estrogen due to the fact that low testosterone levels stimulate the production of LH, which in turn stimulates the aromatase in Leydig cells to produce large amounts of estrogens. Additionally, there is the peripheral conversion of adrenal androgens to estrogens, which helps the misbalance of estrogens to androgens ratio in favor of estrogens.

In secondary hypogonadism, the mechanism of developing gynecomastia is much simpler since the underproduction of gonadotropins results in downregulation of testosterone production in the testes while the aromatization process of adrenal androgens remains undisturbed, producing normal amounts of estrogens (Derkacz et al., 2011).

C. Exogenous or Acquired Causes

Environmental Gynecomastia

Environmental gynecomastia is a very interesting category since it is caused by estrogen excess acquired from the patient's environment. There are synthetic or natural chemical compounds, which imitate estrogen's function and are called xenoestrogens.

Table 3. Causes of hypogonadism

Primary Hypogonadism	Secondary Hypogonadism
5a-reductase deficiency	Hypopituitarism – Hyperprolactinemia
Androgen insensitivity syndrome	Pituitary lesions
Congenital anorchia	Idiopathic secondary hypogonadism
Hemochromatosis	Severe or chronic illness
Klinefelter syndrome	Kallmann syndrome
Viral Orchitis	Prader Willi syndrome
Testicular trauma/ torsion	Drug use (opiates, alcohol abuse)

These xenohormones have weak estrogen function but are capable of triggering gynecomastia and affecting other aspects of a person's health (Andersson and Skakkebaek, 1999).

There are several routes of taking up these substances either through diet, occupational activities or domestic products. The consumption of plants or meat, which contain xenoestrogens in large quantities and for a long time, could contribute to the development of gynecomastia. For example, the phytoestrogen genistein in soy and 8-prenulnaringenin in hops are believed to be able to trigger gynecomastia, although experiments on primates do not validate the effect of soy in the development of gynecomastia (Derkacz et al., 2011; Martinez et al.,2008; Wood et al., 2006). Soy consumption is considered safe up to 300 mg per day since amounts larger than that have been reported to cause gynecomastia (Messina, 2010). Other cases of gynecomastia are associated with the consumption of needle teas and Chinese 'Dong Quai' tablets, which contain pulverized roots of Chinese Angelica ((Derkacz et al., 2011). Athletes are known to develop gynecomastia after the consumption of Burra Gokharu (tribulis terrestris) as an alternative to steroids (Derkacz et al., 2011). Occupational or domestic exposure to xenoestrogens is another reason for environmental gynecomastia. Such substances are found in fodder, plant-protection, paint, and cleaning products. Another category is the indirect exposure to hygiene and beauty products, which contain estrogen additives, substances with estrogen function or lavender and tea tree oil (contains weak estrogenic and anti-androgenic function). Characteristic of this category is the gynecomastia developed in prepubertal boys after indirect exposure to creams applied by their mothers. Finally, there is another case of environmental gynecomastia, which is not based on the excess of estrogens acquired from products but on the effect of substances with antiandrogenic function. Such effect was described on Haitian refugees who were exposed to phenothin, which has antiandrogenic function and it was contained in the spray used to treat lice infestation (pediculosis) in these men (Brody and Loriaux, 2003).

Lifestyle Gynecomastia

Lifestyle gynecomastia is preferred on occasions where the patient overdoes certain habits for a long time,often observed during vacation time. The first report of vacational gynecomastia was in the early 1990s and it was attributed to consumption of large amounts of alcohol and poultry (Heufelder et al., 1992). The effect of alcohol consumption in developing gynecomastia might be associated with the phytoestrogens that are contained in specific kinds of alcohol, the decreased production of testosterone due to testicular dysfunction or the increased peripheral conversion of adrenal androgens to estrogens (Derkacz et al., 2011). As for the poultry, it is believed that substances with estrogen function are contained in the fodder and through consumption concentrate in the animal meat and then passonto the male person. Another lifestyle habit associated with gynecomastia is smoking of marijuana and the use of other narcotic substances, for example amphetamines (Derkacz et al., 2011). Specifically, marijuana is believed to act as a phytoestrogen and interferes with estrogen receptors (Barros and Sampaio, 2012).

Medication Related Gynecomastia

Medication related gynecomastia is a well-known side effect of chronic treatment of a certain disease with a specific medication. In the United States, more than 300 pharmaceutical substances have been associated with the potential development of gynecomastia. The percentage of medication related gynecomastia in this disease is quite high, reaching up to 25% in some studies (Eckman and Dobs, 2008). The categories of drugs that are associated with gynecomastia have a wide range from antibiotics, chemotherapeutics, hormonal, retroviral, psychiatric drugs to pharmaceutical substances used for cardiovascular and gastric diseases. The common parameter in the underlying mechanism of these drugs is the chronic usage of such treatments. The main pathogenetic mechanism is based on directly or indirectly disrupting the estrogen-to-androgen ratio in favor of the numerator. However, according to the nature of the pharmaceutical substance, different combinations of drugs can lead to the same result. For example, there are substances with estrogenic function, and othersthat compete with estrogen connecting to SHBG, increase aromatase function, have antiandrogenic function or increase PRL secretion. Table 4 describes some of the drugs that are related with gynecomastia.

Spironolactone is one of the most well-known pharmaceutical substances related to gynecomastia. It is a steroid antimineralocorticoid with a complex mechanism of triggering gynecomastia. Spironolactone increases the peripheral conversion of testosterone to estradiol, diminishes testosterone production, dislodges testosterone from SHBG enabling degradation of this hormone, and blocks the function of the androgen receptor (Cuhaci et al., 2014).

Calcium channel blockers such as nifedipine and verapamil are also well known substances related to gynecomastia. These two have the highest correlation with this disease while diltiazem (another calcium channel blocker) has the lowest (Cuhaci et al., 2014). Although the exact mechanism is not well defined for most of these substances, there is the exception of verapamil, which is believed to trigger gynecomastia via hyperprolactinemia (Fearrington et al., 1983).

Another category of drugs related with gynecomastia is the H2 receptor antagonist family, which decreases the basic and triggered gastric secretion. It is used in gastric disorders such as peptic ulcers and gastroesophageal reflux disease. Cimetidine is known to trigger gynecomastia by increasing the levels of active estradiol. On the other hand, ranitidine is the family member with the lowest correlation to gynecomastia.

Table 4. Medical substances associated with gynecomastia

	Medical Substance	Category	Disease	Therapeutic mechanism of action	Mechanism of developing gynecomastia
ANTIANDROGENS	Bicalutamide, Flutamide	Non-steroidal antiandrogen	Prostate cancer	AR antagonist, increased degradation of AR	Anti-androgenic properties
	Cyproterone	Steroidal antiandrogen, progestin, antigonadotropin	Prostate cancer	AR antagonist, Inhibition of LH secretion	Anti-androgenic properties, Inhibition of testosterone synthesis
	Goserelin, Leuprorelin, Buserelin	Antihormonal agent	Prostate cancer, breast cancer, endometriosis	GnRH/ LHRH agonist with initial flare	Inhibition of testosterone synthesis
	Finasteride, Dutasteride	5a-reductase inhibitor	Benign prostatic hyperplasia	Blocks conversion of testosterone to dihydrotestosterone	Reduction of serum dihydro-testosterone
ANTIBIOTICS-ANTIRETROVIRAL DRUGS	Isoniazid	Antibiotic	Tuberculosis	Inhibits synthesis of mycobacterial cell wall	Unknown mechanism
	Ketoconazole	Imidazole antifungal	Fungal infection	Disrupts permeability of cell membrane	Plural mechanisms resulting in an E/A increase
	Metronidazole	Nitroimidazole antibiotic	Bacterial, protozoal infection	Blocks DNA synthesis	Unknown-possibly inhibiting testosterone synthesis or action
	HAART (Indinavir)	AntiHIV therapy	HIV therapy	Blocks HIV1/2 protease	Unknown
CARDIOLOGICAL-ANTIHYPERTENSIVE DRUGS	Nifedipine, Verapamil, Diltiazem	Calcium channel blocker	Hypertension, angina	Blocks membrane calcium channels	Unknown- possibly via hyper-prolactinemia
	Captopril, Enalapril	ACE inhibitor	Hypertension	Antagonistic inhibitor of ACE	Unknown

Table 4. (Continued)

	Medical Substance	Category	Disease	Therapeutic mechanism of action	Mechanism of developing gynecomastia
	Digoxin	Cardiac glycoside	Atrial fibrillation / flutter	Na+/K+ pump inhibitor mainly in myocardium	Estrogenic properties
	Glyceryl trinitrate, Isosorbide dinitrate, Isosorbide-5-mononitrate	Organic nitrate esters (Nitrates)	Angina pectoris, myocardial infarction, congestive heart failure	Vascular smooth muscles relaxation and dilation of coronary vessels	Unknown
	Prazosin, Tamsulosin, Doxazosin	Alpha-blocker	Hypertension, Benign blood pressure	Selective blockade of α1 receptors → vasodilation	Unknown
	Spironolactone	Diuretic	Hypertension	Aldosterone receptor antagonist	↑ conversion of testosterone to estradiol, ↑ degradation oftestosterone,blocks the function of AR
HORMONES	Anabolic steroids	Anabolic androgenic steroids	Athletes, Body Building	Androgen receptor agonist	Estrogens predomination within cycles of administration
	Estrogens	Estrogenic steroids or xenoestrogens	Prostate cancer	Estrogen receptor agonist	Estrogenic properties

	Medical Substance	Category	Disease	Therapeutic mechanism of action	Mechanism of developing gynecomastia
PSYCHIATRIC DRUGS	Haloperidol	Butyrophenone derivate antipsychotic	Schizophrenia, acute psychosis, mania etc.	Inverse dopamine receptor antagonist	Hyperprolactinemia
	Diazepam	Benzodiazepine → Positive allosteric modulator of GABA type A receptor	Anxiety, panic attack, insomnia, seizures, etc.	Promotes binding of GABA to GABA receptor	↑ concentration of SHBG
	Imipramine, Clomipramine, Amitriptyline	Tricyclic antidepressants	Depressive disorders	Modifying serotonin reuptake regulation	Unknown
GASTRIC DISORDERS	Cimetidine, Ranitidine	Antihistamine drug of acid related disorder	Peptic ulcers, gastroesophageal reflux disease	Histamine H2-receptor antagonist	↑ levels of active estradiol
	Omeprazole	Proton pump inhibitor	Peptic ulcers, gastroesophageal reflux disease, dyspepsia, Zollinger-Ellison syndrome	Proton pump inhibitor	Unknown
	Metoclopramide	Antiemetic, gastroprokinetic drug	Vomiting, nausea, gastric emptying in gastroparesis	Dopamine D2 receptor antagonist	Hyperprolactinemia
	Domperidone	Antiemetic, gastroprokinetic drug	Vomiting, nausea, gastric emptying in gastroparesis	Peripheral Dopamine D2 and D3 receptor antagonist	Hyperprolactinemia
HYPOLIPIDE-MIC DRUGS	Atorvastatin, Rosuvastatin	Statin	Dyslipidemia, Cardiovascular disease	Competitive inhibitor of HMG-CoA reductase	Inhibition of testosterone synthesis, ↓ serum testosterone levels
	Fenofibrate	Fibrate	Hypercholesterolemia, mixed dyslipidemia	Activating PPARa	Unknown
CHEMOTHE-RAPY	Methotrexate	Antifolate drug	Cancer treatment	Inhibiting dihydrofolate reductase	Unclear but may due to induced increased breast sensitivity to estrogen
	Alkylating Drugs	Antineoplasmic agent	Cancer treatment	Attaching an alkyl group to guanine base of DNA	Gonadal (Leydig cells) dysfunction

Table 4. (Continued)

		Medical Substance	Category	Disease	Therapeutic mechanism of action	Mechanism of developing gynecomastia
OTHERS		Vincristine, Vinblastine	Vinca alkaloid	Cancer treatment	Inhibiting assembly of microtubule structure	Unclear, maybe due to gonadal (Leydig cells) dysfunction
		Theophylline	Xanthine family drug	Respiratory diseases: chronic obstructive pulmonary disease, asthma	Competitive nonselective phosphodiesterase inhibitor, nonselective adenosine receptor antagonist	Unknown
		Penicillamine	Chelating agent	Rheumatoid arthritis, Wilson's disease, cystinuria, scleroderma	Act as chelating agent for excretion of copper, cystrine	Unknown
		Phenytoin	Hydantoin–derivative anticonvulsant drug	Complex partial and generalized tonic-clonic seizures	Binding to the inactive form of the sodium channel	↑ concentration of SHBG

AR: Androgen Receptor, LH: Luteinizing Hormone, GnRH: Gonadotropin-Releasing Hormone, LHRH: Luteinizing-Hormone-Releasing Hormone, E/A: Estrogen/ Androgen, HAART: Highly Active Antiretroviral Therapy, GABA: Gamma-Aminobutyric Acid, SHBG: Sex Hormone Binding Globulin, ACE: angiotensin converting enzyme.

Omeprazole is another drug used to treat gastic disorders, which is related with gynecomastia, although there are no sophisticated studies proving that this substance is associated with increased risk of gynecomastia (Cuhaci et al., 2014). Another well-known drug used in gastrointerstinal diseases is metoclopramide and it is associated with the development of gynecomastia. The underlying mechanism is based on increased levels of serum prolactin found after metoclopramide treatment (Madani and Tolia, 1997).

Digoxin is a powerful inotropic drug extracted from the plant foxglove. Except for the effects on cardiac muscle, digoxin also has estrogenic effects and it can be classified as a phytoestrogen since it has structural resemblance with estradiol and can interfere with estrogen receptors (Biggar, 2012). In women, digoxin is related with increased risk of estrogen-sensitive cancers while in men it is associated with gynecomastia (Biggar, 2012; Karnath 2008).

Androgen deprivation therapy for prostate cancer or benign hyperplasia can trigger development of gynecomastia since it disrupts the estrogen-to-androgen balance. The incidence of gynecomastia in these patients can reach 70% for specific treatments (Barros and Sampaio, 2012). Hormonal antiandrogen therapy for prostate cancer contains several different categories of drugs such as luteinizing-releasing hormone agonists (goserelin, leuprolide, buserelin), synthetic estrogens (diethylstilbestrol), and antiandrogens (bicalutamide, flutamide, cyproterone). As for prostate hyperplasia treatment, finasteride (an inhibitor of 5a-reductase) is also associated with the development of gynecomastia.

An interesting mechanism of developing gynecomastia is observed in males using anabolic steroids. The administered testosterone results in a negative feedback of testosterone testicular production. However, the treatment schedule requires cycles of testosterone administration with appropriate free-of-drug time intervals. During the free-of-drug periods the testosterone levels are very low, due to cessation of natural production. Therefore, in these periods estrogens predominate resulting in the development of gynecomastia.

Finally, there is the HIV treatment-related gynecomastia, which is developed in patients undergoing highly active antiretroviral therapy (HAART) for HIV infection (Meercotter, 2010). The exact mechanism is not well-established. The two possible hypotheses are that drugs might have estrogenic function or that recovery of the immune system after treatment improves estrogen availability (Meercotter, 2010).

Miscellaneous Reasons of Gynecomastia

Gynecomastia is associated with several other conditions, which are not defined as diseases but are considered as the causative event of developing gynecomastia such as spinal cord injury, psychological stress, varices of the spermatic cord, and obesity. Spinal cord disorders and especially injuries are known to be associated with gynecomastia in some cases. Although the exact mechanism is not known, it is believed that disorders of diencephalon or disruption of gonadal function might be the causative factor of gynecomastia (Derkacz et al., 2011). Psychological stress has been implicated in some cases as the intriguing event of developing hormonal unbalance favoring the presence of transient gynecomastia. During stressful events, it is believed that cortisol and estrogen are increased and testosterone is decreased within the normal range (Derkacz et al., 2011). Additionally, it is supported that adrenal androgens are increased in response to stress, which subsequently are converted to estrogens (Gooren and Daantje, 1986). As for the effect of varicocele in the development of gynecomastia, it is believed that the testicular dysfunction caused by the varices of the spermatic cord could result in estrogen-to-androgen unbalance favoring the presence of gynecomastia (Castro-Magana et al., 1991). Obesity is associated with two forms of male breast enlargement. Firstly, it is the pseudogynecomastia, which is defined as enlargement of the male breast, exclusively caused by accumulation of adipose tissue without any participation of the mammary gland. Secondly, it is the true gynecomastia, which is connected to obesity through the leptin hormone. Leptin is a polypeptide hormone produced by adipocytes according to the state of their triglyceride reserves (Myers et al., 2010). Although leptin decreases food intake, it is found in high levels in some obese persons. This paradox is attributed to leptin resistance that these persons might have (Myers et al., 2010). Leptin is also associated with estrogen production, since it is able to stimulate aromatase at adipocytes. Additionally, leptin is believed to participate in the pathogenesis of pubertal gynecomastia since it was found at high levels at pubertal patients (Dundar et al., 2005). Therefore, the presence of high levels of leptin in obese persons with leptin resistance could be the underlying cause of true gynecomastia in such patients, due to increased estrogen production through peripheral aromatization (Dickson, 2012).

Prepubertal and Pubertal Pathologic Gynecomastia

Prepubertal gynecomastia is constantly a sign of gynecomastia's pathologic origin. The etiology of this symptom might be a systematic disturbance, a congenital dysfunction of the gonadal organs or an environmental intervention. In early prepuberty, the most common reason is exposure to exogenous estrogens either through cosmetics containing estrogens, which are used by adults of the family, or accidental ingestion of hormonal pills or consumption of estrogen containing food products. One characteristic sign of such an etiology is the strong pigmentation of areolas and nipples. Other causes that might produce systematic disturbances are testicular tumors secreting estrogen (Sertoli or Leydig cell tumors) or β-HCG. Although feminizing adrenal tumors are rare in children, they can be identified as the etiological causein some cases. Another rare reason of prepubertal gynecomastia is the congenital dysfunction of the steroidogenesis machinery,represented by aromatase excess syndrome.

Pubertal gynecomastia is considered as one of the three categories of physiologic gynecomastia, taking into account that it is transient and it will resolve on its own within two years of the onset. Persistent pubertal gynecomastia on the other hand, is categorized to the pathologic gynecomastia and it is defined as the pubertal gynecomastia, which persists after 17 years of age or after two years from the onset of symptoms (Dickson 2012). In such cases, the first reason, which should be investigated, is the use of certain drugs or anabolic steroids. As in prepubertal gynecomastia, other reasons are the administration of exogenous estrogens, testicular or adrenal tumors, and aromatase excess syndrome. Additionally, cases of primary hypogonadism such as Klinefelter syndrome, androgen insensitivity syndrome, and defects of testosterone biosynthesis should be investigated. Finally, there are other systemic diseases, which could result in secondary hypogonadism, which could be the underlying reason of pathologic pubertal gynecomastia.

Genetic Diseases Associated with Gynecomastia

Gynecomastia has a strong genetic background. It is developed in several disorders of sexual hormones or organs derived from chromosomal anomalies, gene mutations, and polymorphisms. Common syndromes such as Klinefelter's and Peutz-Jeghers as well as rare syndromes such as Borjeson-Forssman-Lehmann are described to have gynecomastia as one of the characteristic anomalies. Other disorders related to gynecomastia are the aromatase excess syndrome, Kennedy's disease, and androgen insensitivity syndrome. Finally, there are polymorphisms in genes such as *CYP19*, *ERS2*, and *LEPR,* which are shown to be the causative factor of gynecomastia.

Klinefelter's Syndrome

Klinefelter's syndrome (KS) is the most common cause of male hypogonadism found in 0.2% of general population (Wosnitzer and Paduch, 2013). Gynecomastia is observed in 50 to 80% of patients and it is attributed to primary hypogonadism (Karnath, 2008; Dercacz et al., 2011). KS is caused by meiotic nondisjunction resulting in a 47XXY karyotype with an aberrant X chromosome.

The main characteristics of KS phenotype are micropenis, small testes with spermatogenic and steroidogenic deficiency, infertility, hypergonado-tropic hypogonadism with low levels of testosterone, tall stature, sparse hair in region associated with secondary sex characteristics, gynecomastia, behavioral and learning issues (Wosnitzer and Paduch, 2013; Karnath, 2008). Although the phenotype of KS males is characteristic, there is a wide range of phenotypic variation and most of them are diagnosed during puberty.

The hormonal profile of KS males is in accordance to primary hypogonadism with low testosterone levels, high levels of LH and FSH. Estrogens can be found either in normal values or increased, due to overexpression of aromatase (Wosnitzer and Paduch, 2013; Dercacz et al., 2011). Low testosterone is attributed to testicular dysfunction accompanied by the small size of Leydig cells and loss of germ and Sertoli cells (Wosnitzer and Paduch, 2013).

KS is associated with several other diseases or conditions such as obesity, high levels of estrogens, diabetes mellitus, hypothyroidism, hypoparathy-roidism, growth hormone deficiency, autoimmune diseases and increased risk of breast and germ cell cancer (Wosnitzer and Paduch, 2013). It is the only case of gynecomastia, which is accompanied with increased risk of breast cancer.

Aromatase Excess Syndrome

Aromatase excess syndrome (AEXS) or familial gynecomastia is a genetic disease characterized by increased serum estrogen levels, the presence of gynecomastia and overexpression of the*CYP19A1* gene. It is a rare autosomal dominant disorder caused by heterogenous chromosomal rearrangements.

CYP19A1 gene is located on 15q21.2 locus and it spans 123 kb (Fukami et al., 2012). It consists of 11 noncoding exons 1 and nine coding exons 2-10. Each of the noncoding exons 1 is accompanied by specific promoter regions and it is expressed at different tissues. The main chromosomal rearrangements associated with AEXS are inversions, duplications and deletions. The proposed etiology of these chromosomal events is the presence of specific motifs around the *CYP19A1* gene that are susceptible to rearrangement (Fukami et al., 2012).

The symptoms of this disease are gynecomastia, small testes, tall stature during childhood and short stature in adulthood as well as accelerated bone age (Fukamiet al., 2012;Dercacz et al., 2011). In women, this syndrome is associated with macromastia and increased risk of gynecological cancer (Dercacz et al., 2011).

The hormonal profile of such patients comprises increased estrogen levels and estrogen-to-androgen ratio, low testicular and adrenal androgens levels, normal LH but low FSH levels (Fukami et al., 2012). The main underlying mechanism of gynecomastia in this disease is the increased estrogen-to-androgen ratio favoring the development of the mammary gland.

11β-Hydroxylase and 21-Hydroxylase Deficiencies

Congenital adrenal hyperplasia is a genetic disorder associated with enzymatic defects of the cortisol and aldosterone biosynthesis pathways. The phenotypic variation of this disorder is based on the grade of enzymatic deficiency. Congenital adrenal hyperplasia is mainly attributed to 21-hydroxylase deficiency (90-95% of the cases) and secondly to 11β-hydroxylase deficiency (5-8% of cases; Yoo et al., 2013; Wasniewska et al., 2009). This disorder is also associated with prepurbertal gynecomastia in boys.

Congenital adrenal hyperplasia is caused by defects of enzyme 21-hydroxylase, which converts progesterone to deoxycorticosterone (aldosterone pathway) and 17-hydroxyprogesterone to deoxycortisol (cortisol pathway). On the other hand, 11β-hydroxylase converts deoxycorticosterone to corticosterone (aldosterone pathway) and deoxycortisol to cortisol (cortisol pathway). Deficiencies in these enzymes trigger secretion of ACTH, which in turn results in accumulation of cortisol precursors. Subsequently, enhanced adrenal androgen production promotes virilization of prepubertal girls and feminization of prepubertal boys due to increased peripheral aromatization of androstenedione to estrone (Blackett and Freeman, 1996).

Other important findings of congenital adrenal hyperplasia are hyponatremia and hyperkalemia. Additionally, early pubic hair, phallic enlargement, and advanced skeletal maturation are observed in children. In 11β-hydroxylase deficiencies, hypertension is observed due to increased concentrations of deoxycorticosterone. The 21-Hydroxylase enzyme is encoded by the*CYP21* gene located on the 6p21.3 chromosomal locus, within the HLA histocompatibility complex. Additionally, there is a pseudogene named *CYP21P,*which is in close proximity. The main mutational mechanism of *CYP21*gene is its recombination with the pseudogene *CYP21P* resulting in an inactive *CYP21* gene (Forest, 2004). On the other hand, the 11β-hydroxylase enzyme is encoded by the *CYP11B1* gene, which is located on the 8q22 chromosomal locus close to the aldosterone synthase gene *CYP11B2* (Mornet et al., 1989). The deficiency of this gene is acquired through mainstream mutational mechanisms such as missense, nonsense, spice site mutations and insertions resulting in frame shift changes (Merke et al., 1997; Helmberg et al., 1992).

Peutz-Jeghers Syndrome

Peutz-Jeghers syndrome is an autosomal dominant disorder characterized by multiple gastrointestinal hamartomatous poluposisand mucocutaneous melanin deposition at lips, buccal mucosa, and digits. It is also associated with an increased risk of developing various neoplasms. The gene responsible for Peutz-Jeghers syndrome is *LKB1 (ST11)*, a serine/threonine kinase, located on the 19p13.3 chromosomal locus (Wang et al., 1999).

LKB1 (ST11) gene spans 23 kb and consists of 10 exons of which the first nine are coding regions and the last one is noncoding (Papp et al., 2010). The expressed protein is a tumor suppressor serine/threonine kinase known to phosphorylate thirteen members of the AMP-activated protein kinase family (Zac-Varghese et al., 2014). This kinase contributes to the regulation of cell polarity, cell growth, metabolism, and survival.

The Peutz-Jeghers syndrome is associated with the development of polyps at any position of the gastrointestinal tract with the most common location being the small bowel, colon, stomach, and rectum. The presence of large hamartomatous polyps can result in bowel obstructions. The causative event of Peutz-Jeghers syndrome is germline mutations of the *STK11* gene. Such mutations are found in 70-80% of Peutz-Jeghers syndrome cases and they vary from nonsense mutations to splice-junction alterations, insertionsand deletions, which result in loss of function mutations (Chae and Jeon, 2014).

Gynecomastia in Peutz-Jeghers syndrome is associated with the presence of feminizing calcified Sertoli cell tumors, which are known as large-cell calcifying Sertoli cell tumors (LSCT). These tumors are usually developed in younger patients and are benign when they are accompanied with endocrine function (Lefevre et al., 2006). The main underlying mechanism of developing gynecomastia in such tumors is the overexpression of aromatase, which in turn results in increased levels of circulating estrogens due to peripheral conversion of adrenal androgens and testosterone (Crocker et al., 2014).

Borgeson-Forssman-Lehman Syndrome

Borgeson-Forssman-Lehman Syndrome (BFLS) is a rare syndrome associated with an X-linked partially dominant clinical picture of mental retardation, obesity, hypogonadism, and dysmorphic features. More specifically, the main characteristics of BFLS are epilepsy, microcephaly, coarse facial features, long ears, short stature, obesity, gynecomastia, small genitalia, tapering fingers and shortened toes. In general, affected males show a milder clinical picture than females (Cecz et al., 2006).

The BFLS is attributed to mutations of the *PHF6* gene, which is located on the Xq26.2 chromosomal locus and it is a member of a large family of zinc-finger genes (Lower et al., 2002). It consists of 11 exons and there are two main mRNA isoforms, which differ by the presence or splicing of intron 10 (Lower et al., 2002). The protein is located on the nucleus and it is possibly associated with transcriptional regulation.

The mutations of the*PHF6*gene related to BFLS are missense mutations, deletions or nucleotide changes which result in truncated proteins(Cecz et al., 2006). Most of these mutations are identified within exon 2 to 10. As for the gynecomastia, it is assumed that it develops due to the hypogonadism observed in these patients.

Spinal and Bulbar Muscular Atrophy

Spinal and bulbar muscular atrophy (SPMA), also known as Kennedy's disease, is an X-linked polyglutamine (polyQ) disease, which is characterized by motor neuron degeneration and androgen insensitivity symptoms such as gynecomastia and testicular atrophy. The responsible gene is *AR* (androgen receptor),which is located on Xq12 and it spans over 90 kb. It consists of eight exons and the protein is divided into three major functional domains: the N-terminal domain, the DNA binding domain and the androgen-binding domain. AR is a transcription factor activated by the binding of androgens.

The *AR* gene contains two polymorphic trinucleotide repeat segments encoding glytamine and glycine. Both of these segments are located on the N-terminal region of the protein. The CAG trinucleotide repeat, which is translated to the polyglytamine segment of the protein, is located on exon 1 and it is responsible for the SPMA (Thomas et al., 2006). Normally, this repeat consists of 5 to 35 triplets. On the other hand, SBMA patients are found to have 37 or more triplets in this trinucleotide repeat (Thomas et al., 2006). SBMA is one of the nine polyglytamine (poly Q) neurodegenerative diseases in which the elongated polyQ repeats are believed to be the toxic factor for neuron cells. The main mechanism of polyQ toxicity is based on the misfolding of AR proteins when testosterone binds on this receptor. The misfolded proteins accumulate in the spinal cord motor neurons and muscle cells resulting in degeneration of these cells (Giorgetti et al., 2014). Gynecomastia in these patients is developed in accordance to testicular atrophy, impaired fertility and increased levels of androgens indicating a mild or moderate grade of androgen insensitivity (Dejager et al., 2002).

Androgen Insensitivity Syndrome

Androgen insensitivity syndrome is presented in three forms, the complete, partial and mild androgen insensitivity syndrome. In the complete form, the phenotype of the patient is female while its karyotype is male (XY). This female person has testes, which produce androgens but due to peripheral aromatization, it develops secondary female sexual characteristics. Although there is development of the breast and vagina, there is lack of internal female gonadal organs such as ovaries, fallopian tubes, and uterus (Hughes et al., 2012). In partial androgen insensitivity syndrome, the usual phenotype is male with micropenis, severe hypospadias, and bifid scrotum (Hughes et al., 2012). In mild form, the phenotype is definitely male with problems of infertility and in some cases gynecomastia. Spinal and bulbar muscular atrophy is considered as a subtype of mild androgen insensitivity syndrome.

The androgen insensistivity syndrome is caused by mutations on the *AR* (androgen receptor)gene. In complete and partial forms of this syndrome the missense mutations are distributed throughout the coding region of the protein but mainly at the functional domains of DNA and ligand binding, resulting in loss of function of this receptor (Hughes et al., 2012).

The development of gynecomastia in this syndrome is associated with decreased androgens function regardless of the serum levels of these steroids and on the other hand, the increased estrogens function due to peripheral aromatization of the testicular and adrenal androgens.

Gene Polymorphisms and Gynecomastia

An important part of gynecomastia is classified as idiopathic since there is no obvious etiological factor of triggering mammary gland development and the hormonal levels in these patients are within normal range. However, recent studies associate gynecomastia with specific gene polymorphisms in otherwise normal males. The most well studied gene is *CYP19*, which encodes the aromatase enzyme. So far, more than 80 *CYP19* polymorphisms have been identified and some of them have been associated with estrogen dependent diseases such as breast cancer, endometrial cancer, and others (Ma et al., 2005; Czajka-Oraniec et al., 2008). As for gynecomastia, there are two polymorphisms, which are indicated to result in an increased risk of gynecomastia in men and macromastia in women. The first is a short tandem repeat tetranucleotide (TTTA)n located on intron 4 of the *CYP19*. Men with this microsatellite polymorphism have increased risk of developing gynecomastia (Czajka-Oraniec et al., 2008). The second is a single nucleotide polymorphism (SNP) C/T (rs10046) located on exon 10 3'-UTR (untranslated region). The two alleles are shown to have different aromatase activity with the T proven to have increased function (Kristensen *et al.*, 2000). Therefore, men who have the T allele are associated with having an increased incidence of gynecomastia (Czajka-Oraniec et al., 2008).

Other genes associated with gynecomastia are *ESR2* (Estrogen receptor beta) and *LEPR* (Leptin receptor). Recent studies try to relate polymorphisms of these genes with increased risk of gynecomastia. So far, *ESR2*AluI 1730G>A polymorphism (rs4986938) and LEPRGln223Arg polymorphism (rs1137101) are believed to be triggering factors of gynecomastia in some males (Eren et al., 2014).

References

Anbazhagan, R., Bartek, J., Monaghan, P., Gusterson, B.A. (1991). Growthand development ofthe human infant breast. *Am. J. Anat.*, 192, 407-417.

Andersson, A.M., Skakkebaek, N.E. (1999). Exposure to exogenous estrogens in food: possibleimpact on human development and health. *Eur. J. Endocrinol.*, 140, 477-485.

Andersson, A.M., Toppari, J., Haavisto, A.M., Petersen, J.H., Simell, T., Simell, O., Skakkebaek, N.E. (1998). Longitudinal reproductive hormone profiles in infants: peak ofinhibin B levels in infant boys exceeds levels in adult men. *J. Clin. Endocrinol. Metab.*, 83, 675-681.

Barros, A.C., Sampaio, M.C. (2012). Gynecomastia: physiopathology, evaluation and treatment. *Sao Paulo Med. J.*, 130, 187-197.

Biggar, R.J. (2012). Molecular pathways: digoxin use and estrogen-sensitivecancers--risks and possible therapeutic implications. *Clin. Cancer Res.*, 18, 2133-2137.

Blackett, P.R., Freeman, D.A. (1996). Androstenedione aromatization as a cause of gynecomastia in 11beta-hydroxylase and 21-hydroxylase deficiencies. *Endocr. Pract.*, 2, 90-93.

Brody, S.A., Loriaux, D.L. (2003). Epidemic of gynecomastia among Haitian refugees:exposure to an environmental antiandrogen. *Endocr. Pract.*,9, 370-375.

Castro-Magana, M., Angulo, M., Uy, J. (1991). Elevated serum estradiol associated withincreased androstenedione-testosterone ratio in adolescent males with varicocele and gynecomastia. *Fertil. Steril.*, 56, 515-518.

Chae, H.D., Jeon, C.H. (2014). Peutz-Jeghers syndrome with germline mutation of STK11. *Ann. Surg. Treat. Res.*, 86,325-330.

Chentli, F., Bekkaye, I., Yahiaoui, S., Souidi, S., Fedala, N.S., Azzoug, S. (2013). Feminizingadrenal tumors: Our experience about three cases. *Indian J. Endocrinol. Metab.*, 17, 509-513.

Crocker, M.K., Gourgari, E., Lodish, M., Stratakis, C.A. (2014). Use of Aromatase Inhibitors inLarge Cell Calcifying Sertoli Cell Tumors: Effects on Gynecomastia, GrowthVelocity, and Bone Age. *J. Clin. Endocrinol. Metab.*,jc20142530, [Epubahead of print].

Cuhaci, N., Polat, S.B., Evranos, B., Ersoy, R., Cakir, B. (2014). Gynecomastia: Clinicalevaluation and management. *Indian J. Endocrinol. Metab.*, 18, 150-158.

Czajka-Oraniec, I., Zgliczynski, W., Kurylowicz, A., Mikula, M., Ostrowski, J. (2008). Association between gynecomastia and aromatase (CYP19) polymorphisms. *Eur. J. Endocrinol.,*158, 721-727.

Dandona, P., Rosenberg, M.T. (2010).A practical guide to male hypogonadism in the primarycare setting. *Int. J. Clin. Pract.,* 64, 682-696.

Derkacz, M., Chmiel-Perzyńska, I., Nowakowski, A. (2011). Gynecomastia - a difficultdiagnostic problem. *Endokrynol. Pol.*, 62, 190-202.

Dejager, S., Bry-Gauillard, H., Bruckert, E., Eymard, B., Salachas, F., LeGuern, E.,Tardieu, S., Chadarevian, R., Giral, P., Turpin, G.(2002). A comprehensive endocrinedescription of Kennedy's disease revealing androgen insensitivity linked to CAGrepeat length. *J. Clin. Endocrinol. Metab.*, 87, 3893-3901.

Dickson, G. (2012). Gynecomastia. *Am. Fam. Physician*, 85, 716-722.

Dimitrakakis, C., Bondy, C. (2007). Androgens and the breast. *Breast Cancer Res.*, 11, 212.

Dundar, B., Dundar, N., Erci, T., Bober, E., Büyükgebiz, A. (2005). Leptin levels in boys with pubertal gynecomastia. *J. Pediatr. Endocrinol. Metab.,* 18, 929-934.

Eckman, A., Dobs, A. (2008). Drug-induced gynecomastia. *Expert Opin. Drug Saf.,* 7, 691-702.

Eren, E., Edgunlu, T., Korkmaz, H.A., Cakir, E.D., Demir, K., Cetin, E.S., Celik, S.K. (2014). Genetic variants of estrogen beta and leptin receptors may cause gynecomastia in adolescent. *Gene*, 541, 101-106.

Fearrington, E.L., Rand, C.H. Jr., Rose, J.D. (1983). Hyperprolactinemiagalactorrhea inducedby verapamil. *Am. J. Cardiol.,* 51, 1466-1467.

Forest, M.G. (2004). Recent advances in the diagnosis and management of congenital adrenal hyperplasia due to 21-hydroxylase deficiency. *Hum. Reprod. Update,* 10, 469-485.

Fukami, M., Shozu, M., Ogata, T. (2012). Molecular bases and phenotypic determinants of aromatase excess syndrome. *Int. J. Endocrinol.,* 2012, 584807.

Gécz, J., Turner, G., Nelson, J., Partington, M. (2006). The Börjeson-Forssman-Lehmansyndrome (BFLS, MIM #301900). *Eur. J. Hum. Genet.,* 14, 1233-1237.

Giorgetti, E., Rusmini, P., Crippa, V., Cristofani, R., Boncoraglio, A., Cicardi, M.E.,Galbiati, M., Poletti, A. (2014). Synergic prodegradative activity of Bicalutamide andtrehalose on the mutant androgen receptor responsible for spinal and bulbarmuscular atrophy. *Hum. Mol. Genet.*, pii: ddu419, [Epub ahead of print].

Gooren, L.J., Daantje, C.R. (1986). Psychological stress as a cause of intermittentgynecomastia. *Horm. Metab. Res.,* 18, 424.

Helmberg, A., Ausserer, B., Kofler, R. (1992). Frame shift by insertion of 2 basepairs in codon 394 of CYP11B1 causes congenital adrenal hyperplasia due to steroid 11 beta-hydroxylase deficiency. *J. Clin. Endocrinol. Metab.,* 75, 1278-1281.

Heufelder, A.E., Leinung, M.C., Northcutt, R.C. (1992). Holiday gynecomastia. *Ann. Intern. Med.,* 116, 877.

Howard, B.A., Gusterson, B.A. (2000). Human breast development. *J. Mammary Gland Biol. Neoplasia*, 5, 119-137.

Hughes, I.A., Davies, J.D., Bunch, T.I., Pasterski, V., Mastroyannopoulou, K., MacDougall, J. (2012). Androgen insensitivity syndrome. *Lancet,* 380,1419-1428.

Ismail, A.A., Barth, J.H. (2001). Endocrinology of gynaecomastia. *Ann. Clin. Biochem.,* 38, 596-607.

Javed, A., Lteif, A. (2013). Development of the human breast. *Semin. Plast. Surg.,*27,5-12.

Jayasinghe, Y., Cha, R., Horn-Ommen, J., O'Brien, P., Simmons, P.S. (2010). Establishment ofnormative data for the amount of breast tissue present in healthy children up to two years of age. *J. Pediatr. Adolesc. Gynecol.,* 23,305-311.

Jolicoeur, F. (2005). Intrauterine breast development and the mammary myoepitheliallineage. *J. Mammary Gland Biol. Neoplasia,* 10, 199-210.

Karnath B. (2008). Gynecomastia. *Hospital Physician,* 44, 45-51.

Kristensen, V.N., Harada, N., Yoshimura, N., Haraldsen, E., Lonning, P.E., Erikstein, B., Kåresen, R., Kristensen, T., Børresen-Dale, A.L. (2000). Genetic variants of CYP19 (aromatase) and breast cancer risk. *Oncogene,* 19, 1329-1333.

Lefevre, H., Bouvattier, C., Lahlou, N., Adamsbaum, C., Bougnères, P., Carel, J.C. (2006). Prepubertal gynecomastia in Peutz-Jeghers syndrome: incomplete penetrance in afamilial case and management with an aromatase inhibitor. *Eur. J. Endocrinol.,* 154, 221-227.

Leifke, E., Gorenoi, V., Wichers, C., Von Zur Mühlen, A., Von Büren, E., Brabant, G. (2000). Age-related changes of serum sex hormones, insulin-like growth factor-1 andsex-hormone binding globulin levels in men: cross-sectional data from a healthymale cohort. *Clin. Endocrinol. (Oxf.),*53, 689-695.

Lower, K.M., Turner, G., Kerr, B.A., Mathews, K.D., Shaw, M.A., Gedeon, A.K., Schelley, S., Hoyme, H.E., White, S.M., Delatycki, M.B., Lampe,

A.K., Clayton-Smith, J., Stewart, H., van Ravenswaay, C.M., de Vries, B.B., Cox. B., Grompe, M., Ross, S., Thomas, P., Mulley, J.C., Gécz, J. (2002). Mutations in PHF6 are associated with Börjeson-Forssman-Lehmann syndrome. *Nat. Genet.*, 32, 661-665.

Ma, C.X., Adjei, A.A., Salavaggione, O.E., Coronel, J., Pelleymounter, L., Wang, L., Eckloff,B.W., Schaid, D., Wieben, E.D., Adjei, A.A., Weinshilboum, R.M. (2005). Human aromatase: generesequencing and functional genomics. *Cancer Res.*, 65, 11071-11082.

Madani, S., Tolia, V. (1997). Gynecomastia with metoclopramide use in pediatric patients. *J. Clin. Gastroenterol.*, 24, 79-81.

Martinez, J., Lewi, J.E. (2008). An unusual case of gynecomastia associated with soyproduct consumption. *Endocr. Pract.*, 14, 415-418.

McKiernan, J.F., Hull, D. (1981). Prolactin, maternal oestrogens, and breast development in the newborn. *Arch. Dis. Child.*,56, 770-774.

Meerkotter, D. (2010). Gynaecomastia associated with highly active antiretroviraltherapy (HAART). *J. Radiol. Case Rep.*, 4, 34-40.

Merke, D.P., Tajima, T., Chhabra, A., Barnes, K., Mancilla, E., Baron, J., Cutler, G.B. Jr. (1998). Novel CYP11B1 mutations in congenital adrenal hyperplasia due to steroid 11 beta-hydroxylase deficiency. *J. Clin. Endocrinol. Metab.*, 83, 270-273.

Messina, M. (2010). Soybean isoflavone exposure does not have feminizing effects onmen: a critical examination of the clinical evidence. *Fertil. Steril.*, 93, 2095-2104.

Mornet, E., Dupont, J., Vitek, A., White, P.C. (1989). Characterization of two genes encoding human steroid 11 beta-hydroxylase (P-450(11) beta). *J. Biol. Chem.*, 264, 20961-20967.

Myers, M.G. Jr., Leibel, R.L., Seeley, R.J., Schwartz, M.W. (2010). Obesity and leptin resistance:distinguishing cause from effect. *Trends Endocrinol. Metab.*, 21, 643-651.

Papp, J., Kovacs, M.E., Solyom, S., Kasler, M., Børresen-Dale, A.L., Olah, E. (2010). Highprevalence of germline STK11 mutations in Hungarian Peutz-Jeghers Syndrome patients. *BMC Med. Genet.*,11, 169.

Robinson, G.W., Karpf, A.B., Kratochwil K. (1999). Regulation of mammary gland developmentby tissue interaction. *J. Mammary Gland Biol. Neoplasia*, 4, 9-19.

Schmidt, I.M., Chellakooty, M., Haavisto, A.M., Boisen, K.A., Damgaard, I.N., Steendahl, U., Toppari, J., Skakkebaek, N.E., Main, K.M. (2002). Gender difference in breast tissue size ininfancy: correlation with serum estradiol. *Pediatr. Res.*, 52,682-686.

Thomas, P.S. Jr., Fraley, G.S., Damian, V., Woodke, L.B., Zapata, F., Sopher, B.L., Plymate, S.R., La Spada, A.R. (2006). Loss of endogenous androgen receptor protein accelerates motorneuron degeneration and accentuates androgen insensitivity in a mouse model ofX-linked spinal and bulbar muscular atrophy. *Hum. Mol. Genet.*, 15, 2225-2238.

Turashvili, G., Bouchal, J., Burkadze, G., Kolar, Z. (2005). Mammary gland development and cancer. *Cesk. Patol.*, 41, 94-101.

Wang, Z.J., Churchman, M., Avizienyte, E., McKeown, C., Davies, S., Evans, D.G., Ferguson, A., Ellis, I., Xu, W.H., Yan, Z.Y., Aaltonen, L.A., Tomlinson, I.P. (1999). Germline mutations of the LKB1(STK11) gene in Peutz-Jeghers patients. *J. Med. Genet.,* 36, 365-368.

Wasniewska, M., Arrigo, T., Lombardo, F., Crisafulli, G., Salzano, G., De Luca, F. (2009). 11-Hydroxylase deficiency as a cause of pre-pubertal gynecomastia. *J. Endocrinol. Invest.,* 32, 387-388.

Wood, C.E., Appt, S.E., Clarkson, T.B., Franke, A.A., Lees, C.J., Doerge, D.R., Cline, J.M. (2006). Effects of high-dose soy isoflavones and equol on reproductive tissues in female cynomolgus monkeys. *Biol. Reprod.*, 75, 477-486.

Wosnitzer, M.S, Paduch, D.A. (2013). Endocrinological issues and hormonal manipulation in children and men with Klinefelter syndrome. *Am. J. Med. Genet. C Semin. Med. Genet.,*163C, 16-26.

Yoo, Y., Chang, M.S., Lee, J., Cho, S.Y., Park, S.W., Jin, D.K., Park, H.D. (2013). Genotype-phenotype correlation in 27 pediatric patients in congenital adrenal hyperplasia due to 21-hydroxylase deficiency in a single center. *Ann. Pediatr. Endocrinol. Metab.*, 18, 128-134.

Zac-Verghese, S., Trapp, S., Richards, P., Sayers, S., Sun, G., Bloom, S.R., Reimann, F.,Gribble, F.M., Rutter, G.A. (2014). The Peutz-Jeghers kinase LKB1 suppresses polyp growth fromintestinal cells of a proglucagon-expressing lineage. *Dis. Model Mech.*, pii: dmm.014720.

Zamd, M., Farh, M., Hbid, O., Zabari, M., Benghanem Gharbi, M., Ramdani, B., Zaïd, D., El Abbadi, N., Lalaoui, K., Belhouari, A., Hassan Tahri, E. (2004). Sexual dysfunction among 78 Moroccan male hemodialysis patients: clinical and endocrine study. *Ann. Endocrinol. (Paris),* 65, 194-200.

In: Endocrine Diseases
Editor: Kenneth Hines

ISBN: 978-1-63482-592-4
© 2015 Nova Science Publishers, Inc.

Chapter 3

Clinical and Molecular Solutions to the Puzzling Controversies of Hormone Replacement Therapy

Zsuzsanna Suba[*]
National Institute of Oncology
Surgical and Molecular Tumor Pathology Centre
Budapest, Hungary

Abstract

Menopausal hormone replacement therapy (HRT) and its health outcomes have been the subjects of extensive investigation; the results of these however are highly inconclusive. Today, it is considered that the effect of HRT is a complex pattern of the mysterious mixture of risks and benefits and the use of this therapy is not evaluated as safety prevention for chronic diseases. This conclusion implies the unawareness of the crucial role of estrogens in the surveillance of cellular health based on the

[*] Address: H-1122 Ráth György str. 7-9, Tel: 00 36 1 224 86 00, Fax: 0036 1 224 86 20, email: subazdr@gmail.com

misinterpretation of clinical and experimental results. Estrogens and their receptor system have biologically pivotal role favored by evolution as a means of integration of all cellular functions serving the survival and reproduction of individuals. A unique feature of estrogens is their beneficial safeguard on all privileged healthy cells, while they are capable of recognizing malignant tumor cells and killing them by apoptosis. All previous studies related to women receiving HRT were performed on randomly selected patients, disregarding their risk factors for either insufficient estrogen synthesis or defective estrogen receptor transduction pathways. Recently, the Women's Health Initiative (WHI) Randomized Trials, which examined the effect of HRT on hysterectomised, crudely estrogen deficient women, found that estrogen treatment resulted in striking decreases in breast cancer development. Moreover, after re-analyzing the data of earlier WHI studies, subsets of women without strong family history of breast cancer, exhibited significantly reduced breast cancer incidence attributable to one armed estrogen treatment. At the same time, women with a family history of breast cancer could have inherited defective estrogen receptor signaling and reactive but insufficient hyperestrogenism. The perspectives for successful HRT will be the separation of postmenopausal patients according to their different inclination to breast cancer risk. The appropriate estrogen dosage will be beneficial against breast cancer and for many other aspects of women's health as well.

Introduction

Hormone replacement therapy (HRT) in postmenopausal women has been fairly widespread in the economically developed countries in the past decades. Women were expecting the benefit of reducing cardiovascular risk and bone fractures, as well as improving overall quality of life. HRT supplied excellent possibilities to study the associations between female sexual steroid hormones and tumor incidence. The prevailing concept was that HRT is associated with an increased prevalence of breast and gynecological cancers [1, 2, 3]. At the same time, clinical studies on HRT use in postmenopausal women yielded unexpected, inverse associations with malignancies at several sites [4-9], supporting the beneficial effect of improved hormonal equilibrium against cancer risk.

A collaborative re-analysis was performed on data from 51 epidemiological studies dealing mainly with single estrogen substitution [10]. The overall relative risk for breast cancer was as low as 1.14 when HRT users were compared with never users. The increase in the risk was very small but significant because of the great number of examined cases. Nevertheless, some of the clinical studies failed to identify any association between increased serum estrogen levels and breast cancer [11, 12]. Although HRT was regarded as breast cancer risk factor from 10 studies reviewed, only 5 showed statistically significant positive association between hormone treatment and breast cancer risk whereas, the other 5 studies could not justify this correlation [13].

Today, HRT use is regarded as a risky and debated method for either mitigation of anguishing postmenopausal symptoms or for prevention of chronic diseases. Although the results of HRT-studies are highly controversial, direct correlations between estrogen concentrations and breast cancer risk have been erroneously established and strengthened even by recent publication [14].

Use of natural estrogens is suitable for upregulation of all physiologic cellular mechanisms, including estrogen receptor signaling and DNA-stabilizer processes [15]. The correct results of HRT studies may be achieved by understanding that all known breast cancer risk factors are associated with defective estrogen signaling. Successful counteraction against cancer risk factors requires the harmonized adaptation of exogenous hormone treatment so as to upregulate the defective estrogen signaling of patients.

Milestones on the Route of HRT Studies in the XXIst Century

In 2002, data from the Women's Health Initiative (WHI) hormone replacement therapy trials were published, including more than 161 000 U.S. women aged between 50 and 79 years [16]. Overall health risks exceeded benefits from use of combined estrogen plus progestin for an average 5.2-year follow-up among healthy postmenopausal US women. The results supported increases in breast cancer risk among hormone treated women, leading to a major pendulum swing against HRT use.

Ragaz and his colleagues from Canada reviewed and reanalyzed data from the WHI hormone replacement therapy trials. The authors separated the subsets of women with no strong family history of breast cancer receiving estrogen treatment alone and established a significantly reduced breast cancer incidence. In addition, separated subsets of estrogen treated women without benign breast disease prior to the trial enrollment also had a significantly reduced breast cancer risk [17]. This reanalysis of the WHI results suggests that the mechanisms of breast cancer risk factors in the mixed population of postmenopausal women are not uniform and the systematic selection of homogenous subgroups could lead to correct results [18].

Results of the HRT studies obtained from the WHI randomised trials on postmenopausal women with prior hysterectomy were published in 2004. One armed estradiol treatment was found to be associated with a striking reduction in breast cancer risk [19]. The authors could not explain these unexpected findings and suggested that further research is necessary to clarify the sources of these remarkable results.

Seven years later, after cessation of estrogen treatment, the data of women remaining alive were evaluated again. In the earlier estradiol treated group of hysterectomised women, a persistent tumor protective effect was established [20]. None of the authors recognized that the health derangement of hysterectomy may almost uniformly induce the defective estrogen signaling and cancer risk for both the estrogen treated and untreated control cases. Advantageous homogenization of the tumor risk of women included into this study led to the revelation of an equivocally beneficial anticancer effect of estradiol administration.

Nowadays, the opinions of scientists have been partially changed regarding correlations between appropriate estrogen signaling and human health; however, the overwhelming majority of literary data still supports the carcinogenic capacity of estrogens.

Different Mechanisms May Affect the Risk of Breast Cancer via Deficient Estrogen Signaling

Risk factors for breast cancer are usually evaluated when the tumors are clinically diagnosed. Nevertheless, cell kinetic studies of tumors justified that the clinical appearance of solid breast cancers requires at least a period of 6-8 years or even longer from their initiation to the development of palpable size [21]. All the studies showing direct associations between HRT and breast cancer are based on shorter observational periods. Searching for the etiologic factors of breast cancer is difficult, since harmful effects at the estimated time of first mutation in the past might be more crucial than the momentary findings at the time of clinical diagnosis.

Hormonal imbalance may develop in either premenopausal or postmenopausal women. Nevertheless, cancer initiation in premenopausal cases may be clinically manifested later during their postmenopausal period, as tumor growth may take a long time, depending on the strength of endogenous counteractions.

Age-Related Defects of Estrogen Signaling Affecting the Risk of Breast Cancer

Great hormonal changes occurring during a woman's life might strongly define the inclination to initiate any type of breast cancer including poorly differentiated ER-negative ones [15]. The stronger the hormonal imbalance characterized mainly by hyperinsulinism, hyperandrogenism and low estrogen exposure, the higher the breast cancer risk, particularly for the poorly differentiated types.

Three main phases seem to be particularly dangerous for breast cancer initiation during the life of women [15]. Two of these are crucial periods inducing hormonal and metabolic storms; adolescence (14-18 years) and the perimenopausal phase (45-55 years). Both periods present risks for overall breast cancer initiation if the biologic processes in the background become pathologic. The third, especially risky phase for breast cancer initiation is older age (over 60 years) when the hormonal and metabolic imbalance becomes stronger and the defense mechanisms against cancer initiation are debilitated.

The first challenges for the whole body of girls are *pubertal changes*, since the abrupt somatic and sexual development means a real danger for the development of insulin resistance and the associated imbalance of male-to-female sexual hormone ratio [22, 23]. When a young girl inherits genetic or acquires somatic anomaly; such as glucose intolerance or obesity, overproduction of androgens will develop at the expense of defective estrogen synthesis [24]. This hormonal disturbance may induce insidiously symptom-free ovulatory failure or irregular anovulatory menstrual cycles [25]. In severe cases, polycystic ovarian syndrome (PCOS) develops with defective estrogen signaling and insulin resistance, which is the most prevalent hormonal disease in young women [26].

Adolescent hyperandrogenism is usually preserved till the early thirties and leads to definite or prolonged infertility resulting in nulliparity or delayed childbirth [27, 28]. Low estrogen exposure and androgen excess at young age may provoke anovulatory infertility as well as initiation and even clinical appearance of breast, endometrial and ovarian cancers in premenopause [24, 29]. Thus, reproductive failures and female cancer development have typically common sources; long lasting hyperandrogenism, defective estrogen synthesis associated with insulin resistance.

In healthy premenopausal women, breast cancer development is rare as preserved ovulatory menstrual cycles are protective and even a slightly or moderately defective estrogen synthesis may counteract cancer initiation [24]. However, increasing grades of insulin resistance associated with enhanced severity of sexual hormone imbalance mean high risks for breast cancer development even in young cases and particularly for the initiation of poorly differentiated tumors [15].

In case of mild *hyperinsulinemia* and hyperandrogenism, preserved circulatory female sexual steroid levels and regular menstrual cycles may usually be enough to protect against breast tumor initiation. With aggravation of insulin resistance in young women, the associated moderate decrease in circulating estrogen level may cut off the ovulatory estrogen peak resulting in anovulatory infertility. Even this slightly estrogen deficient milieu may confer preferential risk for breast cancer as well as for endometrial and ovarian malignancies in anovulatory women. These female organs have the highest estrogen demand so as to preserve their structural and functional integrity [24].

Among premenopausal cases, the *metabolic syndrome* is associated with particular increase in the risk for ER-PR- cancers and TNBCs [30] parallel with decreasing estrogen exposure. In young premenopausal cases with *type-2 diabetes*, progressive insulin resistance and blocked aromatase activity inhibit the conversion of androgens to estrogen in both the ovaries and peripheral tissues [31]. Low estrogen exposure is incapable of defending the cellular functions against strong insulin resistance and hyperandrogenism [24, 32, 33] resulting in early initiation and rapid clinical appearance of poorly differentiated, aggressive breast tumors [15].

Artificial cycles created by oral contraceptives (OCs) improves insulin resistance and provides substantial protection against endometrial and ovarian cancer in the endangered anovulatory women [34, 35]. By contrast, the effect of OCs on breast cancer risk seems to be highly controversial. Increased risk was found to be confined to women who have begun pill use as teenagers or who had been pill users for a long time [36]. Conversely, the relative risk was slightly decreased (0.9) for those who had previously used OC [37], and in cases that had used OCs for at least 10 years a markedly reduced risk for ER+ breast cancer was observed [38]. Adequate selection of patients and controls having similar endogenous and familial risk factors should lead to the real evaluation of beneficial OC effect against breast cancer risk [24].

Correlations between OC use and risk for different breast cancer subtypes are even much more controversial in young women. Although OCs may improve the hormonal equilibrium in both healthy and anovulatory women, there are fairly diverse hormonal statuses among OC non user control cases, which may disturb the results concerning breast cancer risk [15, 24].

The second risky period for breast cancer initiation may be the *perimenopausal phase*, when there is a slow or steep decline in ovarian female sexual steroid synthesis and the last menstrual cycle approaches. Breast cancer initiation is relatively frequent in these hormonally challenged women between the ages of 45 and 55 and these tumors are predominantly hormone receptor positive, which is attributed to the inequalities of the decreasing estrogen supply [29].

In perimenopause, breast and other peripheral tissues may exhibit rapid compensatory hormone production for the completion of decreasing ovarian estrogen synthesis in an amount sufficient to kill or differentiate breast tumor cells initiated by chance. In this case menopausal women are generally complaint free and do not require medical help. In further cases, the gradual hormonal adaptation to ovarian senescence is defective and the beginning of tissular estrogen synthesis in the breast is late. This delay may result in tumor initiation, but later the increasing extraovarian estrogen synthesis may promote the differentiation of early cancers [39]. These women, with transitorily insufficient estrogen level frequently have strong menopausal complaints.

Postmenopausal hormone replacement therapy (HRT) is typically associated with highly differentiated, ER positive tumors, which are initiated in the late premenopausal or perimenopausal period of moderate hormonal failure, much earlier than the beginning of hormone treatment [40]. Estrogen administration may help to differentiate the already existing subclinical tumors; however the dose of hormone replacement is not always enough to kill them. The clinical diagnosis is always postmenopausal in case of tumors initiated in the late premenopausal or perimenopausal phase due to the long latency period.

The breast cancer risk of women after hysterectomy may be near uniformly high attributed to the abrupt, shocking estrogen deprivation [29]. A follow up study on hysterectomised cases and controls justified the significantly lower risk of breast cancer in the estrogen-treated group of women [20].

Breast cancers diagnosed *in elderly women over 65*, are typically initiated in the postmenopausal period over 60. These patients are generally non HRT users and exhibit deepening estrogen deficiency and insulin resistance, even a high prevalence of type-2 diabetes and obesity. Both obesity and highly elevated fasting blood glucose level were found to be especially dangerous for mammary malignancies in elderly cases over 65 years of age [41, 42]. There is an increase in the ratio of TNBC among breast cancers in elderly cases, attributed to the low circulatory and tissular estrogen levels, hyperandrogenism and associated insulin resistance. Since women from the elderly population are much fewer than middle aged postmenopausal cases, pooled examinations of breast tumors diagnosed after menopause may give a blurred value with a predominance of hormone receptor positive cases.

Taken together, the risk for breast cancer is directly associated with the grade of defects in the metabolic and hormonal equilibrium during the whole life of women. Although breast cancer may be multicausal, the lack of sufficient estrogen surveillance seems to be crucial risk for the development of mammary tumors in both young and older cases [18].

Correlations between Reproductive Failure, Defective Estrogen Signaling and the Risk of Breast Cancer

Correlations between reproductive capacity and breast cancer risk represent the greatest challenge for epidemiologists for a long time. Revolutionary molecular characterization of breast cancer subtypes yielded further paradigms and contradictions [15].

The apparently controversial correlations between parity and the development of breast cancer subtypes suggested that hormonally mediated factors might be differently or quite inversely related to the development of ER+ and ER- breast cancers [43].

It has been hypothesized that risk for ER^+ breast cancer is directly associated with a women's lifetime exposure to endogenous ovarian hormones; thus parity may strongly reduce the risk by decreasing the number of ovulatory cycles over a lifetime [44, 45]. By contrast, as triple-negative breast cancers are ER-, risk factors operating through hormonal mechanisms are presumed to be less important in the etiology of these tumors as compared with ER^+ cancers [43].

Multiparity in women, and risk for malignancies at several sites exhibit a strong inverse correlation [46-48]. High parity shows tumor protective effect even against the cancers of highly hormone dependent female organs including overall breast cancer, endometrial and ovarian tumors [49]. In anovulatory patients, a significantly decreased overall cancer risk was reported after ovulation induction and in vitro fertilization assisted childbirth, mainly due to a lower than expected incidence of breast cancer [50].

In experimental animals, pregnancy equivalent high estrogen administration could consequently prevent the development of transplanted or chemically induced mammary tumors [51-53]. In ovariectomized, female mice, alcohol consumption and obesity enhanced the growth of experimental mammary tumors, while estrogen supplementation triggered the loss of body fat, improved insulin sensitivity and suppressed tumor growth [54, 55].

Parity and particularly multiparity are associated with a strongly decreased risk of the predominant ER+ breast cancer type [43, 56]. Among parous women, even the number of births was inversely associated with the risk of ER+ breast cancer (HR=0.88) [57] and among women who had at least four pregnancies, a fairly decreased risk of ER+ breast cancer (OR=0.55) was observed [58]. Conversely, TNBC incidence exhibited an apparently unchanged ratio in parous women [57], whereas in certain studies even an increased risk of TNBC was reported in multiparous cases [59, 60]. In a recent study the number of births was found to be directly associated with the risk of TNBC [43].

Nulliparity is generally in correlation with anovulatory disorders, thus these hormone deficient cases may be regarded as opposite extremes as compared with multiparous women [24].

Delayed first childbirth may also be associated with prolonged defective estrogen synthesis and ovulatory failures. Postpubertal sexual hormone imbalances are frequently associated with definite or prolonged fertility disorders resulting in nulliparity or delayed first childbearing [61] and inducing increased overall breast cancer risk among premenopausal women [62, 63].

High overall breast cancer risk in correlation with defective estrogen synthesis and anovulatory disorders justifies the role of physiologic estrogen level in preservation of mammary health [24]. Administration of pregnancy mimicking estrogen and progesterone doses to nulliparous women seems to be a useful strategy for protection against breast cancer [64].

Certain studies suggested that nulliparity plays quite inverse role in the risks of ER+ breast cancer and TNBC as compared with multiparity [65]. Nulliparous status of women was associated with a 35% higher risk of ER+ breast cancer (HR=1.35), whereas with a 39% lower risk for TNBC (HR=0.61) [43]. Delayed first childbirth was also directly associated with risk for ER+ cancers, but showed no remarkable effect on the risk of TNBCs [57].

Considering the apparently contradictory results, if women undertake more childbirth they may be exposed to a stronger risk of developing TNBC, conversely, if they remain nulliparous they are exposed to higher risk for ER+ cancers. So what should they do?

In multiparous women, good fertility associated excellent estrogen signaling and extremely high estrogen levels during pregnancies strongly and equivocally reduce the development of overall breast cancers and the predominant ER+ tumors in particular. A plausible explanation is that estrogen, being the specific ligand for ERs, may preferentially block the development and progression of ER+ cancers. However, its killing capacity against ER- cancers is slower and weaker as the specific tumor receptors are missing. In its complexity, in estrogen rich milieu a fairly decreased number and percentage of ER+ tumors is associated with a moderately decreased number and an unchanged or deceivingly increased percentage of ER- breast cancers [15].

By contrast, in nulliparous hormonally challenged women, the weakness of estrogen surveillance results in enhanced overall breast cancer risk. The insufficient estrogen supply has a defective killing capacity even against the predominant, hormone sensitive ER+ breast cancer cells resulting in an increased number and percentage of surviving ER^+ tumors. The survival possibility for hormonally weakly controlled ER- cancers like TNBCs may disproportionately improve and their raw number may be slightly increased, while the relative number (percentage) decreases [15].

For women being afraid of breast cancer, it is plausible to choose parity either by natural way or by in vitro fertilization, since pregnancy upregulates estrogen signaling and helps to prevent the development of both TNBC and non-TNBC type tumors.

Metabolic Syndrome and Type-2 Diabetes Are Associated with the Defect of Estrogen Signaling and Breast Cancer Risk

Today, it is widely accepted that the higher the grade of insulin resistance with or without obesity in women, the higher the risk for the development of a more aggressive breast cancer [66, 67]. The *metabolic syndrome (MS)* is a phase of insulin resistant state characterized by a quartet of elevated fasting glucose, dyslipidemia, hypertension and visceral obesity [68]. Each of these symptoms alone is a risk factor for cancer and together they mean a multiple risk [69, 70].

MS is associated with increased overall breast cancer risk, higher tumor aggressivity and poorer prognosis [71]. Positive correlations were found between MS and breast cancer incidence, due primarily to positive associations with serum levels of glucose and triglyceride, as well as diastolic blood pressure [72]. Elevated fasting glucose level proved to be a significant risk for breast cancer in both pre- and postmenopausal women [73]. Among breast cancer cases 26% were considered obese, 16% hyperglycemic, 54% hypertensive and 30% dyslipidemic.

In Ireland, MS was established in 39% of all newly diagnosed breast cancer cases and was associated with more aggressive tumor biology. Patients with advanced pathologic stage (II-IV) at diagnosis had MS in 51% of cases, whereas among early stage cases this ratio was only 12% [71]. A meta-analysis of twenty studies estimated a 20% increased risk of breast cancer for women with *type-2 diabetes* [74]. A review of epidemiologic studies on the association between type 2 diabetes and breast cancer risk revealed moderate association appearing to be more consistent among hormonally challenged postmenopausal than premenopausal women [75].

In young premenopausal women a wide range of insulin resistant states may occur from mild hyperinsulinism to diabetes mellitus, which are associated with different stages of androgen excess as well as defective estrogen synthesis [24]. Polycystic ovarian syndrome (PCOS) in young cases is associated with anovulatory infertility and insulin resistance [26] and represents common risk for the cancers of highly hormone dependent breast, endometrium and ovary [76].

In women with PCOS, oral contraceptive (OC) administration improves anovulatory disorders and has favorable impacts on carbohydrate and lipid metabolism as well [34]. OC therapy creates a regular artificial cycle, ameliorates hirsutism and acne and is protective against the development of endometrial carcinoma [35].

In the mildly hyperandrogenic syndromes, only the ovulatory estrogen peak is missing, which results in occult anovulatory infertility and preferential cancer risk for the female organs with high estrogen demand [24]. Nevertheless, the preserved, but slightly defective estrogen level may be enough for the killing or differentiation of randomly initiated breast cancer cells. Accidental failures of estrogen defense in these cases yield biologically milder, ER+ cancer development. Taken together, the lower incidence rate of breast cancers in young cases with low grade insulin resistance may be attributed to the relatively preserved estrogen surveillance [15].

In young women, another extremity of insulin resistance is advanced visceral obesity and/or type-2 diabetes conferring high breast cancer risk attributed to the concomitant hyperinsulinism, hyperandrogenism, defective aromatase activity and a failure of estrogen synthesis [24, 32]. Low estrogen supply cannot counteract the severe dysmetabolism and hyperandrogenism in premenopausal women, which explains the relatively increased incidence rate of poorly differentiated breast cancers, including TNBCs [15].

Postmenopausal aging in women seems to exhibit close correlation with an increased prevalence of MS [77]. The risk of postmenopausal breast cancer was significantly increased in case of women with MS (OR = 1.75) with the risk being much higher above the age of 70 years (OR =3.04). Breast cancer incidence in women diagnosed at or after the age of 65 was strongly associated with highly elevated fasting blood glucose levels (> or =7.0 mmol/l) [42].

MS and type 2 diabetes seem to be preferential risk factors for TNBC as compared with the ER+ breast cancer risk. In a sample of 176 individuals, 58 % of TNBC patients exhibited the comorbid condition of MS as compared with 37% of the non-TNBC cases, using the MS criteria of the National Cholesterol Education Program [67].

Insulin resistant states, such as metabolic syndrome and type-2 diabetes are strong risk factors for breast cancer by several pathways, particularly for the poorly differentiated, ER- tumors like TNBCs. Severe insulin resistance disarms the cellular defense mechanisms by estrogen deprivation and defective estrogen signaling and the strong derangement of estrogen surveillance allows easier escape for ER- tumors. The more advanced the insulin resistance the higher the risk for poorly developed breast cancer [15].

Obesity Mediates Breast Cancer Risk via Defective Estrogen Signaling and Insulin Resistance

Both clinical and experimental evidences prove that obesity, particularly visceral fatty tissue deposition leads to insulin resistance associated with diverse hormonal, metabolic and immunologic alterations mediating breast cancer risk [15, 78, 79].

Distribution of fat deposition is thoroughly affected by male to female sexual steroid equilibrium [80]. In young premenopausal obese women, the overall breast cancer risk is deceivingly moderate, as in the majority of these females adipose tissue deposition is predominantly gluteofemoral resulting in mild insulin resistance counteracted by the preserved hormonal cycle [24]. However, male-like central obesity and severe dysmetabolism in young obese women are associated with hyperandrogenism and a decrease in serum estradiol levels, particularly in the follicular phase of the cycle [81]. Increased obesity-related and PCOS associated breast cancer risk may be attributed particularly to this hormonal imbalance [24, 32].

In postmenopausal estrogen deficient, obese women the regional distribution of fat deposition near uniformly affects the visceral region in close correlation with severe dysmetabolism, estrogen loss and high breast cancer risk [24]. By contrast, HRT use in obese postmenopausal women equivocally reduces the incidence of breast cancer by means of the improvement of hormonal and metabolic balance [82, 83].

Body mass index (BMI) or body weight in kilograms reflects general adiposity and may not correctly refer to correlations among fat distribution, hormonal disorders and overall breast cancer risk in young cases [84]. In certain studies BMI defined obesity was erroneously reported as being inversely correlated with breast cancer risk in premenopausal women [85, 86], which is indicative of the fact that general obesity is not always reliable in the estimation of tumor risk. By contrast, body circumference measurements; such as hip (HC), waist (WC) and waist to hip ratio (WHR) give better information on abdominal fat accumulation and dysmetabolism related cancer risk [87]. Among obese young women, visceral obesity related high WC and WHR values exhibited direct correlations with increased risk for premenopausal breast cancer [88-90].

In young women with central obesity, the defects of estrogen synthesis and anovulatory infertility are strong risk factors for breast cancer; however, similar hormonal disorders are not rare even among control cases with normal body weight [24]. Strict selection of lean control women with healthy sex hormone equilibrium may equivocally justify the health advantage of normal body weight over obesity.

Slight or moderate insulin resistance in obese young women may be associated with still sufficient estrogen signaling capable of killing the majority of developing ER+ tumors, but the more resistant, aggressive ER-cancers may survive, leading to a relative increase in their incidence rate. By contrast, strong insulin resistance in young obese women may counteract the partially preserved estrogen surveillance, which is more advantageous for the survival of ER-PR- tumors and TNBCs. In the meantime, the number of ER+ tumors may increase as well, attributed to the poor suppressive capacity of hormonal forces.

Considering these difficult correlations among obesity type, grade of insulin resistance, level of estrogen surveillance and its different killing capacities in relation to ER+ and ER- cancers, one can understand the deceiving, apparently controversial clinical and epidemiologic findings.

BMI defined general obesity is typically associated with increased TNBC risk, particularly in premenopausal women. In young cases, overweight and obesity seems to be in consistent direct correlation with the development of TNBC and other ER- types of breast tumors [90]. Similarly, obesity and overweight are much more likely among young cases with TNBC as compared with cases with ER+PR+ tumors [91].

The impact of high BMI on ER+, as well as non-TNBC tumors is not uniform, depending on the hormonal status of obese women. In case of a severe defect of hormonal surveillance, the ER+ cancer risk may show somewhat lower increase as compared with ER- ones [92]. By contrast, when the estrogen defense is relatively preserved in obese young cases, ER+ tumor incidence rate may be largely suppressed [93, 94].

Each of the three circumference measurements for abdominal fat (WC, HC and WHR) was statistically significantly associated with increased incidence of ER- breast cancer in premenopausal cases [95]. Hazard ratios of ER- breast cancer for the highest versus lowest quintile of body fat distribution measures were 2.75 for WC, 2.40 for HC and 1.95 for WHR. These correlations justify that central obesity is strongly associated with increased risk for ER- breast cancers. In a further study, only hip circumference was directly associated with increased breast cancer risk [96]. After adjustment for BMI, both ER+PR+ and ER-PR- breast cancers showed directly but differently increased risk with central obesity (HR=1.65 and 2.65 respectively). These remarkable results justify that in premenopausal women, even visceral obesity associated defective estrogen synthesis may be more suppressive for ER+PR+ tumors than ER-PR- ones.

In conclusion, obesity is a multifaceted disease associated with different grades of dangerous dysmetabolism and sexual hormone imbalance promoting breast cancer development. Obesity associated defective estrogen surveillance allows easier escape for steroid receptor negative tumors than for ER+ ones, resulting in conspicuous accumulation of ER- cancers and TNBCs in obese patients.

Poor Natural Light Exposure Confers Increased Breast Cancer Risk for African-American Women via Defective Estrogen Signaling

Population-based data demonstrated that African-American women develop breast cancer at an earlier age, diagnosed in a more advanced stage and exhibit higher incidence rates for poorly differentiated ER- and TNBC types than white American women [56, 97, 98]. TNBC incidence was found to be significantly higher in black women at all ages as compared with white women [99]. Black race was strongly associated with ER⁻PR⁻ tumors as well regardless of HER2 status [56]. Tumor recurrence rate, metastatic spread and mortality are all disadvantageous among black American women as compared with either Caucasian or Asian groups in America [98, 100-102].

Epidemiologic results suggest that poor light exposure in northern regions is a marked cancer risk factor for their inhabitants, for women in particular [103]. Among countries leading in the rank of female overall cancer morbidity in Europe, northern regions are conspicuously highly represented, such as; Denmark, Iceland, Norway and Sweden [104]. The risk of developing breast cancer is significantly high in Northern America and Europe, while being fairly low in Asia and Africa. Incidence and mortality rates of breast cancer are five times higher in the United States than in Japan [105].

Dark skinned immigrants were found to have an excessive cancer risk as compared with the natives of northern adoptive countries and the age at breast cancer diagnosis was found to be earlier [106, 107]. Excessive cancer risk, rapid progression of poorly differentiated cancers and worse prognosis in black skinned American women may be conferred by poor natural light exposure and increased melatonin synthesis mediated by their high pigmentation [103].

Nowadays, melatonin is regarded as an anticancer agent, presumably being protective against hormone dependent tumors attributed to its antiestrogenic impacts [108, 109]. Results from the Nurses' Health Study cohort added substantial supports to a deceivingly inverse association between melatonin levels and breast cancer risk [110]. Melatonin does indeed suppress the estrogen signaling pathways, as it interferes with the activation of nuclear ERs [111]. Melatonin also inhibits the expression and activity of aromatase enzymes, which are responsible for estrogen synthesis and presumably for the progression of ER+ breast cancers [112, 113]. Nevertheless, the well documented antiestrogenic effects of melatonin administration do not justify its protective effect against cancers of the highly hormone dependent female organs. By contrast, excessive melatonin exposure seems to be rather carcinogenic conferred by the associated defective estrogen signaling, insulin resistance, hypothyroidism and vitamin D deficiency [103].

The increased prevalence of anovulatory disorders and early natural menopause before age 40 in African-American women are manifest due to ovarian failure and are associated with a higher rate of all-cause and cancer-specific mortality [114]. Both infertility and ovarian failure are high risk factors for breast cancer in young women, being congruent with the health disadvantage of African-American women [103]. Melatonin excess in young tumor-free African-American women is associated with obesity, hyperinsulinism, and high free testosterone level resulting also in an increased breast cancer risk [115, 116]. African-American women with breast cancer exhibit the metabolic syndrome, type-2 diabetes and central obesity more frequently than white cases with similar tumors [117, 118].

A population based study revealed wide-spread hypothyroidism among African-American women as compared with whites [119]. As melatonin administration suppresses the thyroid function in animal experiments and clinical examinations [120, 121], disproportional hypothyroidism in black skinned American women may also be attributed to their low light exposure. In a prospective study, hypothyroidism and low FT4 values exhibited direct correlation with increased breast cancer risk [122]. Correlations between the epidemiology of vitamin D deficiency, cancer incidence and mortality were studied in the United States [123]. The African-American population showed evidence of particularly widespread vitamin D deficiency. This observation suggests that adequate vitamin D replacement may be an important measure for reduction of race related health disparities including breast cancer incidence [124, 125].

In conclusion, the racial disadvantage of black skinned American women in the incidence, progression and outcome of breast cancers may largely be attributed to their defective estrogen signaling and further hormonal disturbances associated with insufficient light exposure.

BRCA Gene Mutations Induce High Breast Cancer Risk by Defective Estrogen Signaling

Inherited mutations in BRCA1 or BRCA2 genes predispose to breast, ovarian, and other cancers. Their ubiquitously expressed protein products are implicated in processes fundamental to all cells, including DNA repair and recombination, checkpoint control of cell cycle, and transcription [126]. BRCA gene mutations lead to a defect of DNA double-strand break repair through homologous recombination. Disruption of BRCA proteins in mutation carriers can induce susceptibility to specific types of cancer [127].

Incidence of hereditary breast and ovarian cancers reveals close correlation with BRCA mutations [128]. BRCA1/BRCA2 mutations are responsible for 3-8% of all breast cancer cases, whereas for 30-40% of familial cases. Ten percent of patients with ovarian cancer have a genetic predisposition. About 80% of families with a history of ovarian cancer have mutation in the BRCA1, while 15% in the BRCA2 genes. These correlations suggest strong parallelism between cancer initiations of the breast and ovaries as these organs have similarly high estrogen demand and are fairly vulnerable in case of defective estrogen signaling [29].

Among women with germline BRCA1 mutation near 50% of breast cancers is triple negative presenting with a high grade histologically [129, 130]. Among women with breast cancer, TNBC was established in 57.1% of BRCA1-mutation positive and in 23.3% of BRCA2-mutation positive cases, whereas in only 13.8% of BRCA-negative women [131].

Strong correlation between BRCA mutations and high TNBC risk proposes certain mediators between germline mutations and the risk for poorly differentiated breast cancers. All justified risk factors for breast cancer development seem to be in close correlation with estrogen loss or defective estrogen signaling as well as further associated hormonal disorders. The question arises, whether BRCA mutations may lead to breast cancer and preferentially TNBC development by the defect of estrogen signaling or by quite different pathways.

In BRCA1 gene deficient human ovarian cancer cells, estradiol-mediated transcriptional activity of ERs exhibited a relative decrease [132], while ERα showed an unexpected ligand independent transcriptional activity that was not observed in BRCA1-proficient cells [133]. Increased estrogen independent and defective estrogen dependent stimulations of ERs in BRCA1-deficient tumor cells suggest that high cancer risk may be attributed to the defect of ligand activated ER signal. Ligand independent activation of ERα in tumor cells seems to be a compensatory mechanism of omnipotent estrogen signaling in emergency situations. Excessive estrogen administration emerges as a breakthrough of the blockage of ligand activated ER signaling in BRCA mutation carriers.

Correlations between BRCA1 mutation and low response to fertility treatments were examined, as both germline mutations in BRCA genes and anovulatory infertility are associated with high susceptibility for breast and ovarian cancers [134]. In BRCA1 mutation positive women, the low response rate of ovaries to fertility treatment was significantly increased (33.3%) as compared with BRCA1 mutation negative patients (3.3%). These results support that BRCA1 mutations are associated with defective estrogen signaling reflected by increased rate of ovulatory failure.

In women with BRCA1/2 mutation, earlier age at natural menopause (under the age of 40) was observed significantly more frequently than among unaffected cases (p<0.001) [135, 136]. The high risk of premature ovarian failure among BRCA1/2 carriers reflects the disturbances in estrogen synthesis or estrogen receptor signaling pathways. Disorders of estrogen signaling may at least partially confer the risk of tumors associated with BRCA1/2 mutation [24, 33].

Hyperestrogenism (71.7 pg/ml) was observed in BRCA2 mutation carrier patients as compared with the estrogen levels of women with BRCA1 mutations (45.5 pg/ml) and cases without BRCA mutation (38.5 pg/ml) [137]. Estrogen overproduction may be a contraregulatory effect against defective estrogen signaling in BRCA2 mutation carriers mediating their markedly lower cancer risk compared with the high risk of BRCA1 mutation carriers. These observations justify the possibility of breast cancer prevention by high dose estrogen administration in BRCA1/2 mutation cases.

In BRCA gene mutation carriers, the elevated estrogen levels associated with high parity, with artificial hormonal cycle created by oral contraceptives and estrogen administration may decrease the high cancer risk. Parity in BRCA1 mutation carriers significantly reduced the risk for ovarian cancer [138], moreover, the risk was reduced with each additional full-term pregnancy in women with germline mutation [139]. Furthermore, parity with its highly elevated estrogen level also seemed to be protective against TNBC, similarly like against the predominant ER^+ tumors [58].

Use of oral contraceptives (OCs) was found to highly reduce the risk of ovarian cancers in women with both BRCA1 (OR: 0.56) and BRCA2 mutations (OR: 0.39) [139]. Ovarian cancer risk decreased with each year of long term contraceptive use in women carrying BRCA1 or BRCA2 mutations [140]. Protective effect of OC was established as a chemoprevention against ovarian cancers in young women with BRCA mutations; whereas the OC associated risk of breast cancer in BRCA mutation carriers seemed to be heterogeneous with inconsistent results [141]. Nevertheless, the use of OCs for at least 12 months was associated with strongly decreased breast cancer risk for BRCA1 mutation carriers (OR: 0.22), but not for cases with BRCA2 mutation [142].

Consumption of phytoestrogen-rich foods such as soy emerged as preventive measure against breast cancer. Soy consumption may be beneficial in early life before puberty or during adolescence, according to results of immigrant and epidemiological studies [143]. In animal experiments, prepubertal administration of 17β-estradiol reduced the later risk of breast cancer by inducing a persistent up-regulation of BRCA1 gene [144].

Defective estrogen synthesis and/or disorders in estrogen receptor signaling play significant roles in the development of diverse insulin resistant states [33, 145]. In BRCA mutation carrier women, breast cancer development is frequently associated with high BMI and type-2 diabetes [146, 147]. These observations justify the close correlation between defective estrogen signaling and insulin resistance in the development of breast cancer [32].

In conclusion, BRCA1 and BRCA2 mutations seem to increase the breast cancer risk particularly that of ER-negative subtypes by defective estrogen signaling. Upregulation of these defective genes by means of increased estradiol or phytoestrogen exposure may be a promising measure against mammary carcinogenesis.

Conclusion

Tumor-free postmenopausal women may schematically be categorized into different groups according to the grade of their endogenous inclination for breast cancer development. Such grouping is very important because the diversely endangered cases occurring by chance in the big populations of either hormone treated or untreated cases may lead to many confusions in HRT studies. Moreover, further changes in exogenous cancer risk factors or endogenous mechanisms of women may additionally disturb the settings for examiners in long term HRT studies.

In the first group of postmenopausal women, there are neither known nor unknown breast cancer risk factors. These women have good interplay between estrogen signaling and DNA-stabilizer mechanisms even after menopause, and will thus remain equally tumor-free if they are hormone treated or remain untreated.

In postmenopausal women with slightly defective estrogen signaling and DNA-defense mechanisms, usual doses of one-armed estradiol substitution may achieve the entire disappearance of highly ER-positive early breast cancers before their arrival at a clinically diagnosable phase. In the untreated group of such patients, tumor-free cases may be predominant, while sporadic tumors may occur in cases in which additional risk factors are present.

In the third group, of estrogen deficient postmenopausal cases, insulin resistance, particularly associated with obesity or diabetes, is in correlation with decreased estrogen and elevated androgen levels, which are high risk factors for breast cancer. In these estrogen deficient cases, the usual dose of hormone substitution may be either sufficient or insufficient for tumor arrest, depending on the depth of estrogen deficiency. In the similarly estrogen deficient cases of the untreated group, breast cancer may occasionally develop, particularly in association with central obesity and diabetes.

In a further group of estrogen deficiency, the aromatase CYP19-gene may be mutant and consequently, the defective estrogen synthesis is aggravated in the postmenopausal phase. Depending on the loss of estrogen synthesis, in either uniformly treated or non-treated patients, breast cancer may develop.

In postmenopausal women with different grades of ESR1-gene mutation, estrogen resistance endangers the signaling and DNA-stability. The circulating estrogen level is usually reactively increased within the low range of hormone supply in ageing women. At young age, the genetic defect of ERs may be counteracted by intense estrogen synthesis, while the postmenopausal decline in estrogen concentration may manifest the defect of estrogen signaling. In cases presenting mild ESR1 gene defect, the usual HRT dose may be enough, resulting in a tumor-free life, while in cases with uncompensated serious ER-defect breast cancer may develop in either the HRT user or non-user group.

In BRCA1-mutation carrier postmenopausal women with ER signaling defect, the moderately increased estrogen concentration may dangerously decline with ageing and the usual dose of estrogen substitution is not enough for tumor prevention. In BRCA2-mutation carriers, the initial high aromatase activity maintains a higher estrogen production and better estrogen signaling, consequently resulting in a lower breast cancer incidence. In postmenopausal, hormonally challenged cases however, this defensive effect is exhausted. In BRCA1/2 mutation carriers, breast cancer may develop almost equally in either the treated or non-treated groups of HRT studies.

The effect of uniform HRT-use may be either effective or insufficient for cancer prevention depending on the activity of individual genome-stabilizer capacity in women, and on the presence of further risk factors for breast cancer. In the HRT-user group of postmenopausal women, who need to get help against their complaints, the occurrence of breast cancer could possibly be attributed to the insufficient dose of preventive estrogen administration instead of the carcinogenic capacity of estrogen.

Among non-HRT user women, the range of defective estrogen signaling and DNA-safeguarding capacities as well as other carcinogenic risk factors is similarly wide. These complaint-free untreated women may also have hidden defects in the interactions between DNA-safeguarding systems and estrogen signaling. Non-HRT user women without exogenous estrogenic upregulation of their defense mechanisms may also be prone to breast cancer development if the cancer risk factors are strong enough.

Considering the wide range of possibilities for genome instability and counteractive defensive mechanisms, it would be a miracle to receive realistic results on randomly selected populations of uniformly treated and untreated women in large HRT-studies.

References

[1]   La Vecchia C, Brinton LA, McTiernan A. Menopause, hormone replacement therapy and cancer. *Maturitas.* 39:97-115, 2001.

[2]   Diamanti-Kandarakis E. Hormone replacement therapy and risk of malignancy. *Curr. Opinion Obstet. Gynecol.* 16:73-78, 2004.

[3]   Fernandez E, Gallus S, Bosetti C, Franceschi S, Negri E, La Vecchia C. Hormone replacement therapy and cancer risk: a systematic analysis from a network of case-control studies. *Int. J. Cancer.* 105:408-412, 2003.

[4]   Ettinger B, Friedman GD, Bush T, Quesenberry CP Jr. Reduced mortality associated with long-term postmenopausal estrogen therapy. *Obstet. Gynecol.* 87:6-12, 1996.

[5]   Grodstein F, Clarkson T, Manson J. Understanding the divergent data on postmenopausal hormone therapy. *N. Engl. J. Med.* 348:645-650, 2003.

[6]   Olsson H, Bladström AM, Ingvar C. Are smoking-associated cancers prevented or postponed in women using hormone replacement therapy? *Obstet. Gynecol.* 102:565-570, 2003.

[7]   Rodriguez C, Feigelson HS, Deka A, Patel AV, Jacobs EJ, Thun MJ, Calle EE. Postmenopausal hormone therapy and lung cancer risk in the Cancer Prevention Study II Nutrition Cohort. *Cancer Epidemiol. Biomark. and Prev.* 17:655-660, 2008.

[8]   Camargo MC, Goto Y, Zabaleta J, Morgan D, Correa P, Rabkin CS. Sex hormones, hormonal interventions and gastric cancer risk: a meta-analysis. *Cancer Epidemiol Biomarkers Prev.* 21(1):20-38, 2012.

[9]   McGrath M, Michaud DS, De Vivo I. Hormonal and reproductive factors and the risk of bladder cancer in women. *Am. J. Epidemiol.* 163:236-244, 2006.

[10]   Collaborative Group on Hormonal Factors in Breast Cancer. Collaborative reanalysis of data from 51 epidemiological studies of 52 705 women with breast cancer and 108 411 women without breast cancer. *Lancet.* 350:1047-1059, 1997.

[11]   Garland CF, Friedlander NJ, Barrett-Conner E, Khaw KT. Sex hormones and postmenopausal breast cancer: a prospective study in an adult community. *Am. J. Epidemiol.* 135:1220-1230, 1992.

[12]   Wysowski KK, Comstock GW, Helsing KJ, Lau HL. Sex hormone levels in serum in relation to the development of breast cancer. *Am. J. Epidemiol.* 125:791-799, 1987.

[13]   Pike M, Bernstein L, Spicer D. Exogenous hormones and breast cancer risk. In: Neiderhuber J (ed). *Current Therapy in Oncol. BC Decker*, St. Louis, MO. pp.292-302, 1993.

[14]   Colditz GA, Bohlke K. Priorities for the primary prevention of breast cancer. *CA Cancer J. Clin.* 2014; 64(3):186-94.

[15] Suba Z. Triple-negative breast cancer risk in women is defined by the defect of estrogen signaling: preventive and therapeutic implications. *Onco Targets Ther.* 2014; 7:147–164.

[16] Rossouw JE, Anderson GL, Prentice RL, LaCroix AZ, Kooperberg C, Stefanick ML et al. Risks and benefits of estrogen plus progestin in healthy postmenopausal women: principal results From the Women's Health Initiative randomized controlled trial. *JAMA.* 2002; 288(3):321-33.

[17] Ragaz J, Shakeraneh S. Estrogen prevention of breast cancer: A critical review. In: Suba Z. Ed. Estrogen Prevention for Breast Cancer. Chapter 6. New York, Nova Science Publishers Inc., 2012.

[18] Suba Z. Diverse pathomechanisms leading to the breakdown of cellular estrogen surveillance and breast cancer development: new therapeutic strategies. *Drug Design Devel Ther.* 2014; 8: 1381-1390.

[19] Anderson GL, Limacher M, Assaf AR, Bassford T, Beresford SA, Black H et al. Effects of conjugated equine estrogen in postmenopausal women with hysterectomy: the Women's Health Initiative randomized controlled trial. JAMA. 2004;291(14):1701-12.

[20] LaCroix AZ, Chlebowski RT, Manson JE, Aragaki AK, Johnson KC, Martin L, *et al.* Health outcomes after stopping conjugated equine estrogens among postmenopausal women with prior hysterectomy. A randomized controlled trial. JAMA 2011; 305(13): 1305-14.

[21] Spratt JS, Meyer JS, Spratt JA. Rates of growth of human solid neoplasms: part I. *J. Surg. Oncol.* 60:137-146, 1995.

[22] Baer HJ, Colditz GA, Willett WC, Dorgan JF. Adiposity and sex hormones in girls. *Cancer Epidemiol. Biomarkers Prev* 16(9): 1880-8, 2007.

[23] Stoll BA. Teenage obesity in relation to breast cancer risk. *Int. J. Obes Relat Metab Disord* 22(11): 1035-40, 1998.

[24] Suba Z. Circulatory estrogen level protects against breast cancer in obese women. *Recent Pat Anticancer Drug Discov.* 8(2):154-67, 2013.

[25] Polson DW, Wadsworth J, Adams J et al. Polycystic ovaries: a common finding in normal women. *Lancet* 1:870-872, 1988.

[26] Bloomgarden ZT. Second World Congress on the Insulin Resistance Syndrome: Mediators, pediatric insulin resistance, the polycystic ovary syndrome, and malignancy. *Diabetes Care* 28(8): 1821-1830, 2005.

[27] Apter D, Vihko R. Endocrine determinants of fertility: serum androgen concentrations during follow-up of adolescents into the third decade of life. *J. Clin. Endocrinol. Metab.* 71(4): 970-4, 1990.

[28] Sturgeon SR, Potischman N, Malone KE, Dorgan JF, Daling J, Schairer C, Brinton LA. Serum levels of sex hormones and breast cancer risk in premenopausal women: a case-control study (USA). *Cancer Causes Control.* 15(1):45-53, 2004.

[29] Suba Z. Common soil of smoking-associated and hormone-related cancers: estrogen deficiency. *Oncol. Rev.* 4:73-87, 2010.

[30] Davis AA, Kaklamani VG. Metabolic syndrome and triple-negative breast cancer: a new paradigm. *Int. J. Breast Cancer.* 2012:809291. doi: 10.1155/2012/809291, 2012

[31] Stamataki KE, Spina J, Rangou DB, Chlouverakis CS, Piaditis GP. Ovarian function in women with non-insulin dependent diabetes mellitus. *Clin. Endocrinol. (Oxf)* 45(5): 615-21, 1996.

[32] Suba Z. Interplay between insulin resistance and estrogen deficiency as co-activators in carcinogenesis. *Pathol. Oncol. Res.* 18(2): 123-33, 2012.

[33] Suba Z. Low estrogen exposure and/or defective estrogen signaling induces disturbances in glucose uptake and energy expenditure. *J. Diabetes Metab* 4:22:272-278, 2013.

[34] ESHRE Capri Workshop Group. Ovarian and endometrial function during hormonal contraception. *Hum. Reprod.* 16(7): 1527-35, 2001.

[35] Diamanti-Kandarakis E, Baillargeon J-P, Iuorno MJ, Jakubowicz DJ, Nestler JE.A Modern Medical Quandary: Polycystic Ovary Syndrome, Insulin Resistance, and Oral Contraceptive Pills. *J. Clin. Endocrinol & Metab* 88(5): 1927-1932, 2003.

[36] Deligeoroglou E, Michailidis E, Creatsas G. Oral contraceptives and reproductive system cancer. *Ann. NY Acad. Sci.* 997: 199-208, 2003.

[37] Marchbanks PA, Jill A. McDonald JA, Wilson HG, Folger SG et al. Oral Contraceptives and the Risk of Breast Cancer. *New Engl. J. Med.* 346:2025-2032, 2002.

[38] Bernstein L, Lacey JV Jr. Receptors, associations and risk factor differences by breast cancer subtypes: positive or negative? *J. Natl. Cancer Inst* doi: 10.1093/jnci/djr046. 2011.

[39] Suba Zs. Discovery of estrogen deficiency as common cancer risk factor for highly and moderately estrogen dependent organs. In: Ed. Suba Zs. Estrogen prevention for breast cancer. Nova Science Publishers Inc. New York. 2013, pp. 1-22.

[40] Dietel M, Lewis MA, Shapiro S. Hormone replacement therapy: pathobiological aspects of hormone-sensitive cancers in women relevant to epidemiological studies on HRT: a mini-review. *Human Reprod.* 20: 2052-2060, 2005.

[41] La Vecchia C, Negri E, Franceschi S, Talamini R, Bruzzi P, Palli D, *et al.* Body mass index and postmenopausal breast cancer: an age specific analysis. *Br. J. Cancer* 75(3): 441-4, 1997.

[42] Rapp K, Schroeder J, Klenk J, Ulmer H, Concin H, Diem G, Oberaigner W, Weiland SK: Fasting blood glucose and cancer risk in a cohort of more than 140,000 adults in Austria. *Diabetologia* 49: 945-952, 2006.

[43] Phipps AI, Chlebowski RT, Prentice R, McTiernan A, Wactawski-Wende J, Kuller LH, Adams-Campbell LL, Lane D, Stefanick ML, Vitolins M, Kabat GC, Rohan TE, Li CI. Reproductive history and oral contraceptive use in relation to risk of triple-negative breast cancer. *J. Natl. Cancer Inst.* 103(6): 470-7, 2011.

[44] Key TJ. Hormones and cancer in humans. *Mutat Res.* 333(1-2): 59-67, 1995.

[45] den Tonkelaar I, de Waard F. Regularity and length of menstrual cycles in women aged 41-46 in relation to breast cancer risk: results from the DOM-project. *Breast Cancer Res. Treat* 1996; 38(3): 253-8.

[46] Wolpert BJ, Amr S, Ezzat S, Saleh D, Gouda I, Loay I, *et al.* Estrogen exposure and bladder cancer risk in Egyptian women. *Maturitas* 67(4): 353-7, 2010.

[47] Teras LR, Patel AV, Rodriguez C, Thun MJ, Calle EE. Parity, other reproductive factors, and risk of pancreatic cancer mortality in a large cohort of U.S. women. *Cancer Causes and Control* 16(9): 1035-40, 2005.

[48] Bosetti C, Negri E, Franceschi S, Conti E, Levi F, Tomei F. Risk factors for oral and pharyngeal cancer in women: a study from Italy and Switzerland. *Br. J. Cancer* 82(1): 204-7, 2000.

[49] Britt K, Ashworth A, Smalley M. Pregnancy and the risk of breast cancer. *Endocrine-Related Cancer* 14(4): 907-33, 2007.

[50] Källén B, Finnström O, Lindam A, Nilsson E, Nygren KG, Olausson PO. Malignancies among women who gave birth after in vitro fertilization. *Hum. Reprod..* 26(1):253-8, 2011.

[51] Lay YC, Hamazaki K, Yoshizawa K, Kawanaka A, Kuwata M, Kanematsu S et al. Short-term pregnancy hormone treatment of N-methyl-N-nitrosourea-induced mammary carcinogenesis in relation to fatty acid composition of serum phospholipids in female Lewis rats. *In vivo* 24(4): 553-60, 2010.

[52] Holcomb VB, Hong J, Núñez NP. Exogenous estrogen protects mice from the consequences of obesity and alcohol. *Menopause.* 19(6):680-90, 2012.

[53] Rajkumar L, Kittrell FS, Guzman RC, Brown PH, Nandi S, Medina D. Hormone-induced protection of mammary tumorigenesis in genetically engineered mouse models. *Breast Cancer Res.* 9(1):R12, 2007.

[54] Hong J, Holcomb VB, Kushiro K, Núñez NP. Estrogen inhibits the effects of obesity and alcohol on mammary tumors and fatty liver. *Int. J. Oncol.* 39(6): 1443-53, 2011.

[55] Nkhata KJ, Ray A, Dogan S, Grande JP, Cleary MP. Mammary tumor development from T47-D human breast cancer cells in obese ovariectomized mice with and without estradiol supplements. *Breast Cancer Res. Treat.* 114(1): 71-83, 2009.

[56] Trivers KF, Lund MJ, Porter PL, Liff JM, Flagg EW, Coates RJ, Eley JW. The epidemiology of triple-negative breast cancer, including race. *Cancer Causes Control.* 20(7):1071-82, 2009.

[57] Phipps AI, Malone KE, Porter PL, et al. Reproductive and hormonal risk factors for postmenopausal luminal, HER-2-overexpressing, and triple-negative breast cancer. *Cancer* 113(7):1521–1526, 2008.

[58] Ma H, Wang Y, Sullivan-Halley J, Weiss L, Marchbanks PA, Spirtas R, Ursin G, Burkman RT, Simon MS, Malone KE, Strom BL, McDonald JA, Press MF, Bernstein L. Use of four biomarkers to evaluate the risk of breast cancer subtypes in the women's contraceptive and reproductive experiences study. *Cancer Res.* 70(2): 575-87, 2010.

[59] Millikan RC, Newman B, Tse CK, et al. Epidemiology of basal-like breast cancer. *Breast Cancer Res Treat.* 109(1): 123–139, 2008.

[60] Xing P, Li J, Jin F. A case-control study of reproductive factors associated with subtypes of breast cancer in Northeast China. *Med. Oncol.* 27(3): 926–931, 2010.

[61] Velentgas P, Daling JR. Risk factors for breast cancer in younger women. *J. Natl. Cancer Inst. Monogr* (16): 15-24, 1994.

[62] Opdahl S, Alsaker MD, Janszky I, Romundstad PR, Vatten LJ. Joint effect of nulliparity and other breast cancer risk factors. *Br. J. Cancer* 105(5): 731-6, 2011.

[63] Newcomb PA, Trentham-Dietz A, Hampton JM, Egan KM, Titus-Ernstoff L, Warren Andersen S, *et al.* Late age at full term birth is strongly associated with lobular breast cancer. *Cancer* 117(9): 1946-56, 2011.

[64] Tsubura A, Uehara N, Matsuoka Y, Yoshizawa K, Yuri T. Estrogen and progesterone treatment mimicking pregnancy for protection from breast cancer. *In Vivo.* 22(2):191-201, 2008.

[65] Yang XR, Chang-Claude J, Goode EL, Couch FJ, Nevanlinna H, Milne RL, Gaudet J. Associations of breast cancer risk factors with tumor subtypes: a pooled analysis from the Breast Cancer Association Consortium studies. *J. Natl. Cancer Inst.* 103(3): 250-63, 2011.

[66] Davison Z, de Blacquière GE, Westley BR, May FE. Insulin-like growth factor-dependent proliferation and survival of triple-negative breast cancer cells: implications for therapy. *Neoplasia.* 13(6): 504-15, 2011.

[67] Maiti B, Kundranda MN, Spiro TP, Daw HA. The association of metabolic syndrome with triple-negative breast cancer. *Breast Cancer Res. Treat.* 121(2): 479-83, 2010.

[68] Reaven GM. Insulin resistance, cardiovascular disease, and the metabolic syndrome: How well do the emperor's clothes fit? *Diabetes Care* 2004; 27(4): 1011-1012.

[69] Cowey S, Hardy RW. The metabolic syndrome. A high risk state for cancer? *Am. J. Pathol.* 169(5): 1505-22, 2006.

[70] Doyle SL, Donohoe CL, Lysaght J, Reynolds JV. Visceral obesity, metabolic syndrome, insulin resistance and cancer. *Proc. Nutr. Soc.* 71(1): 181-9, 2012.

[71] Healy LA, Ryan AM, Carroll P, Ennis D, Crowley V, Boyle T, *et al.* Metabolic syndrome, central obesity and insulin resistance are associated with adverse pathological features in postmenopausal breast cancer. *Clin. Oncol. (R Coll Radiol)* 22(4): 281-8, 2010.

[72] Kabat GC, Kim M, Chlebowski RT, Khandekar J, Ko MG, McTiernan A, *et al.* A longitudinal study of the metabolic syndrome and risk of postmenopausal breast cancer. *Cancer Epidemiol. Biomarkers Prev.* 18(7): 2046-53, 2009.

[73] Sieri S, Muti P, Claudia A, Berrino F, Pala V, Grioni S, Abagnato CA, Blandino G, Contiero P, Schunemann HJ, Krogh V. Prospective study on the role of glucose metabolism in breast cancer occurrence. *Int. J. Cancer* 130(4):921-9, 2012.

[74] Larsson SC, Mantzoros CS, Wolk A. Diabetes mellitus and risk of breast cancer: a meta-analysis. *Int. J. Cancer.* 121(4):856-62, 2007.

[75] Xue F, Michels KB. Diabetes, metabolic syndrome, and breast cancer: a review of the current evidence. *Am. J. Clin. Nutr.* 86(3):s823-35, 2007.

[76] Pierpoint T, McKeigue PM, Isaacs AJ, Wild SH, Jacobs HS. Mortality of women with polycystic ovary syndrome at long-term follow-up. *J. Clin. Epidemiol.* 51(7): 581-6, 1998.

[77] Schneider JG, Tompkins C, Blumenthal RS, Mora S. The metabolic syndrome in women. *Cardiol. Rev.* 14(6): 286-91, 2006.

[78] Donohoe CL, Doyle SL, Reynolds JV. Visceral adiposity, insulin resistance and cancer risk. *Diabetol. Metab. Syndr.* 3: 12, 2011.

[79] Rose DP, Vona-Davis L. Interaction between menopausal status and obesity in affecting breast cancer risk. *Maturitas* 66(1): 33-8, 2010.

[80] Poehlman ET, Toth MJ, Gardner AW. Changes in energy balance and body composition at menopause: a controlled longitudinal study. *Ann. Intern Med.* 123(9): 673-5, 1995.

[81] Potischman N, Swanson CA, Siiteri P, Hoover RN. Reversal of relation between body mass and endogenous estrogen concentrations with menopausal status. *J. Natl. Cancer Inst.* 88(11): 756-8, 1996.

[82] Morimoto LM, White E, Chen Z, Chlebowski RT, Hays J, Kuller L, *et al.* Obesity, body size and risk of postmenopausal breast cancer: the Women's Health Initiative (United States). *Cancer Causes Control* 13(8): 41-51, 2002.

[83] Ritte R, Lukanova A, Berrino F, Dossus L, Tjønneland A, Olsen A et al. Adiposity, hormone replacement therapy use and breast cancer risk by age and hormone receptor status: a large prospective cohort study. *Breast Cancer Res.* 14:R76, 2012.

[84] Huang Z, Willett WC, Colditz GA, Hunter DJ, Manson JE, Rosner B, Speizer FE, Hankinson SE. Waist circumference, waist:hip ratio, and risk of breast cancer in the Nurses' Health Study. *Am. J. Epidemiol.* 150(12): 1316-24, 1999.

[85] Franceschi S, Favero A, La Vecchia C, Barón AE, Negri E, Dal Maso L, *et al.* Body size indices and breast cancer risk before and after menopause. *Int. J. Cancer* 67(2): 181-6, 1996.

[86] Kotlyarevska K, Wolfgram P, Lee JM. Is waist circumference a better predictor of insulin resistance than body mass index in U.S. adolescents? *J. Adolesc. Health.* 49(3): 330-3, 2011.

[87] Sonnenschein E, Toniolo P, Terry MB, Bruning PF, Kato I, Koenig KL, *et al.* Body fat distribution and obesity in pre- and postmenopausal breast cancer. *Int. J. Epidemiol.* 28(6): 1026-31, 1999.

[88] Connolly BS, Barnett C, Vogt KN, Li T, Stone J, Boyd NF. A meta-analysis of published literature on waist-to-hip ratio and risk of breast cancer. *Nutr. Cancer.* 44(2):127-38, 2002.

[89] Harvie M, Hooper L, Howell AH. Central obesity and breast cancer risk: a systematic review. *Obes Rev.* 4(3): 157-73, 2003.

[90] Rose DP, Vona-Davis L. Influence of obesity on breast cancer receptor status and prognosis. *Expert Rev. Anticancer Ther* 9(8): 1091-101, 2009.

[91] Kwan ML, Kushi LH, Weltzien E, Maring B, Kutner SE, Fulton RS, Lee MM, Ambrosone CB, Caan BJ. Epidemiology of breast cancer subtypes in two prospective cohort studies of breast cancer survivors. *Breast Cancer Res* 11(3): R31, 2009.

[92] Vona-Davis L, Rose DP, Hazard H, Howard-McNatt M, Adkins F, Partin J, Hobbs G. Triple-negative breast cancer and obesity in a rural Appalachian population. *Cancer Epidemiol. Biomarkers Prev.* 17(12): 3319-24, 2008.

[93] Suzuki R, Orsini N, Saji S, Key TJ, Wolk A. Body weight and incidence of breast cancer defined by estrogen and progesterone receptor status--a meta-analysis. *Int. J. Cancer.* 124(3): 698-712, 2009.

[94] Yang X, Chang-Claude J, Gode E, Couch F, Nevanlinna H, Milne R et al. Analysis of breast cancer risk factors by expression of tumor markers: results of 34 studies in the Breast Cancer Association Consortium (BCAC). *Cancer Res.* 70(8): Suppl 1, 2010.

[95] Harris HR, Willett WC, Terry KL, Michels KB. Body fat distribution and risk of premenopausal breast cancer in the Nurses' Health Study II. *J. Natl. Cancer Inst.* 103(3): 273-8, 2011.

[96] Fagherazzi G, Chabbert-Buffet N, Fabre A, Guillas G, Boutron-Ruault MC, Mesrine S, Clavel-Chapelon F. Hip circumference is associated with the risk of premenopausal ER-/PR- breast cancer. *Int. J. Obes (Lond).* 36(3): 431-9, 2012.

[97] Amirikia KC, Mills P, Bush J, Newman LA. Higher population-based incidence rates of triple-negative breast cancer among young African-American women : Implications for breast cancer screening recommendations. *Cancer* 117(12):2747-53, 2011.

[98] Amend K, Hicks D, Ambrosone CB. Breast cancer in African-American women: differences in tumor biology from European-American women. *Cancer Res.* 66: 8327-30, 2006.

[99] Stead LA, Lash TL, Sobieraj JE, Chi DD, Westrup JL, Charlot M, Blanchard RA, Lee JC, King TC, Rosenberg CL. Triple-negative breast cancers are increased in black women regardless of age or body mass index. *Breast Cancer Res.* 11(2): R18, 2009.

[100] Stark A, Stapp R, Raghunathan A, Yan X, Kirchner HL, Griggs J et al. Disease-free probability after the first primary ductal carcinoma in situ of the breast: a comparison between African-American and White-American women. *Breast Cancer Res. Treat* 131:561-70, 2012.

[101] Holmes L Jr, Opara F, Hossain J. A five-year breast cancer-specific survival disadvantage of African American women. *Afr. J. Reprod. Health* 14:195-200, 2010.

[102] DeSantis C, Naishadham D Jemal A. Cancer statistics for African Americans, 2013. *CA: A Cancer Journal for Clinicians* 63(3): 151-166, 2013.

[103] Suba Z. Light deficiency confers breast cancer risk by endocrine disorders. *Recent Pat Anticancer Drug Discov.* 7(3): 337-44, 2012.

[104] Otto Sz. Cancer epidemiology in Hungary and the Béla Johan National Program for the Decade of Health. *Pathol. Oncol. Res.* 9:126-130, 2003.

[105] Montag A, Kumar V. The female genital system and breast. Chapter 19. In: Kumar V, Abbas AK, Fausto N, Mitchell RN. Eds. Robbins basic pathology, 8th Ed. Philadelphia, Saunders Elsevier, pp. 711-50, 2007.

[106] Mousavi SM, Sundquist J, Hemminki K. Nasopharyngeal and hypopharyngeal carcinoma risk among immigrants in Sweden. *Int. J. Cancer* 127:2888-92, 2010.

[107] Hemminki K, Mousavi SM, Sundquist J, Brandt A. Does the breast cancer age at diagnosis differ by ethnicity? A study on immigrants to Sweden. *Oncologist* 16:146-54, 2011.

[108] Viswanathan AN, Schernhammer ES. Circulating melatonin and the risk of breast and endometrial cancer in women. *Cancer Lett.* 281:1-7, 2009.

[109] Sánchez-Barceló EJ, Cos S, Mediavilla MD, Martinez-Campa C, González A, Alonso-Gózález C. Melatonin-estrogen interactions in breast cancer. *J. Pineal Res.* 38:217-22, 2005.

[110] Schernhammer ES, Hankinson SE. Urinary melatonin levels and postmenopausal breast cancer risk in the nurses' health study cohort. *Cancer Epidemiol. Biomarkers Prev.* 18(1): 74–79, 2009.

[111] Cos S, Gonzalez A, Martínez-Campa C, Mediavilla MD, Alonso-González C, Sanchez Barceló EJ. Estrogen signaling pathway: a link between breast cancer and melatonin oncostatic actions. *Cancer Detect Prev* 30:118-28, 2006.

[112] Gonzalez A, Cos S, Martinez-Campa C, Alonso-Gonzalez C, Sanchez-Mateos S, Mediavilla MD. Selective estrogen enzyme modulator actions of melatonin in human breast cancer cells. *J. Pineal Res.* 45:86-92, 2008.

[113] Knower KC, To SQ, Takagi K, Miki Y, Sasano H, Simpson ER, Clyne CD. Melatonin suppresses aromatase expression and activity in breast cancer associated fibroblasts. *Breast Cancer Res. Treat* 132(2):765-71, 2012.

[114] Li S, Rosenberg L, Wise LA, Boggs DA, Lavalley M, Palmer JR. Age at natural menopause in relation to all-cause and cause-specific mortality in a follow-up study of US black women. *Maturitas*. pii: S0378-5122(13)00108-4, 2013.

[115] Seo D-C, Torabi MR. Racial/ethnic differences in body mass index, morbidity and attitudes toward obesity among U.S. adults. *J. Natl. Med. Assoc.* 98(8): 1300–1308, 2006.

[116] Falkner B, Sherif K, Sumner A, Kushner H. Hyperinsulinism and sex hormones in young adult African Americans. *Metabolism* 48:107-12, 1999.

[117] Rose DP, Haffner SM, Baillargeon J. Adiposity, the metabolic syndrome, and breast cancer in African-American and white American women. *Endocr. Rev.* 28:763-77, 2007.

[118] Sarkissyan M, Wu Y, Vadgama JV. Obesity is associated with breast cancer in African-American women but not Hispanic women in South Los Angeles. *Cancer* 117:3814-23, 2011.

[119] Boucai L, Surks MI. Reference limits of serum TSH and free T4 are significantly influenced by race and age in an urban outpatient medical practice. *Clin. Endocrinol. (Oxf)* 70:788-93, 2009.

[120] Vriend J, Bertalanffy FD, Ralcewicz TA. The effects of melatonin and hypothyroidism on estradiol and gonadotropin levels in female Syrian hamsters. *Biology of Reproduction* 36:719-728, 1987.

[121] Bellipani G, Bianchi P, Pierpaoli W, Bulian D, Ilyia E. Effects of melatonin in perimenopausal women and menopausal women: a randomized and placebo controlled study. *Exp. Gerontol.* 1987; 36:297-310, 1987.

[122] Kuijpens JL, Nyklictek I, Louwman MW, Weetman TA, Pop VJ, Coebergh JW. Hypothyroidism might be related to breast cancer in post-menopausal women. *Thyroid* 15:1253-9, 2005.

[123] Giovanucci E. The epidemiology of vitamin D and cancer incidence and mortality: a review (United States). *Cancer Causes Control* 16:83-95, 2005.

[124] Harris SS. Does vitamin D deficiency contribute to increased rates of cardiovascular disease and type 2 diabetes in African Americans? *Am. J. Clin Nutr* 93:1175S-78S, 2011.

[125] Grant WB, Peiris AN. Possible role of serum 25-hydroxyvitamin D in black-white health disparities in the United States. *J. Am. Med. Dir. Assoc.* 11:617-28, 2010.

[126] Venkitaraman AR. Cancer susceptibility and the functions of BRCA1 and BRCA2. *Cell* 108: 171–182, 2002.

[127] Farmer H, McCabe N, Lord CJ, Tutt AN, Johnson DA, Richardson TB, Santarosa M, Dillon KJ, Hickson I, Knights C, Martin NM, Jackson SP, Smith GC, Ashworth A. Targeting the DNA repair defect in BRCA mutant cells as a therapeutic strategy. *Nature.* 434:917-21, 2005.

[128] Lux MP, Fasching PA, Beckmann MW. Hereditary breast and ovarian cancer: review and future perspectives. *J. Mol. Med. (Berl* 84:16–28,) 2006.

[129] Lakhani SR, Van De Vijver MJ, Jacquemier J, Anderson TJ, Osin PP, McGuffog L, Easton DF. The pathology of familial breast cancer: predictive value of immunohistochemical markers estrogen receptor, progesterone receptor, HER-2, and p53 in patients with mutations in BRCA1 and BRCA2. *J. Clin. Oncol.* 20(9): 2310-8, 2002.

[130] Lee E, McKean-Cowdin R, Ma H, Spicer DV, Van Den Berg D, Bernstein L, Ursin G. Characteristics of triple-negative breast cancer in patients with a BRCA1 mutation: results from a population-based study of young women. *J. Clin. Oncol.* 29(33): 4373-80, 2011.

[131] Atchley DP, Albarracin CT, Lopez A, Valero V, Amos CI, Gonzalez-Angulo AM, Hortobagyi GN, Arun BK. Clinical and pathologic characteristics of patients with BRCA-positive and BRCA-negative breast cancer. *J. Clin. Oncol.* 26(26): 4282-8, 2008.

[132] Zheng L, Annab LA, Afshari CA, Lee WH, Boyer TG. BRCA1 mediates ligand-independent transcriptional repression of the estrogen receptor. *Proc. Natl. Acad. Sci. USA* 98(17): 9587-92, 2001.

[133] Fan S, Ma YX, Wang C, Yuan RQ, Meng Q, Wang JA, Erdos M, Goldberg ID, Webb P, Kushner PJ, Pestell RG, Rosen EM. Role of direct interaction in BRCA1 inhibition of estrogen receptor activity. *Oncogene.* 20(1): 77-87, 2001.

[134] Oktay K, Kim JY, Barad D, Babayev SN. Association of BRCA1 mutations with occult primary ovarian insufficiency: a possible explanation for the link between infertility and breast/ovarian cancer risks. *J. Clin. Oncol.* 28(2): 240-4, 2010.

[135] Lin WT, Beattie M, Chen LM, Oktay K, Crawford SL, Gold EB, Cedars M, Rosen M. Comparison of age at natural menopause in BRCA1/2 mutation carriers with a non-clinic-based sample of women in northern California. *Cancer* 119(9): 1652-9, 2013.

[136] Finch A, Valentini A, Greenblatt E, Lynch HT, Ghadirian P, Armel S, Neuhausen SL, Kim-Sing C, Tung N, Karlan B, Foulkes WD, Sun P,

Narod S; Hereditary Breast Cancer Study Group. Frequency of premature menopause in women who carry a BRCA1 or BRCA2 mutation. *Fertil Steril* 99(6): 1724-8, 2013.

[137] Kim J, Oktay K. Baseline E(2) levels are higher in BRCA2 mutation carriers: a potential target for prevention? *Cancer Causes Control.* 24(3): 421-6, 2013.

[138] McLaughlin JR, Risch HA, Lubinski J, Moller P, Ghadirian P, Lynch H, Karlan B, Fishman D, Rosen B, Neuhausen SL, Offit K, Kauff N, Domchek S, Tung N, Friedman E, Foulkes W, Sun P, Narod SA; Hereditary Ovarian Cancer Clinical Study Group. Reproductive risk factors for ovarian cancer in carriers of BRCA1 or BRCA2 mutations: a case-control study. *Lancet Oncol.* 8(1): 26-34, 2007.

[139] Antoniou AC, Rookus M, Andrieu N, Brohet R, Chang-Claude J, Peock S et al. Reproductive and hormonal factors, and ovarian cancer risk for BRCA1 and BRCA2 mutation carriers: results from the International BRCA1/2 Carrier Cohort Study. *Cancer Epidemiol. Biomarkers Prev.* 18(2):601-10, 2009.

[140] Whittemore AS, Balise RR, Pharoah PD, Dicioccio RA, Oakley-Girvan I, Ramus SJ et al. Oral contraceptive use and ovarian cancer risk among carriers of BRCA1 or BRCA2 mutations. *Br. J. Cancer.* 91(11): 1911-5, 2004.

[141] Cibula D, Zikan M, Dusek L, Majek O. Oral contraceptives and risk of ovarian and breast cancers in BRCA mutation carriers: a meta-analysis. *Expert Rev. Anticancer Ther.* 11(8):1197-207, 2011.

[142] Milne RL, Knight JA, John EM, Dite GS, Balbuena R, Ziogas A et al. Oral contraceptive use and risk of early-onset breast cancer in carriers and noncarriers of BRCA1 and BRCA2 mutations. *Cancer Epidemiol Biomarkers Prev.*14(2):350-6, 2005.

[143] Adlercreutz HJ. Phytoestrogens and breast cancer. *Steroid Biochem. Mol. Biol.* 83(1-5): 113-8, 2002.

[144] Cabanes A, Wang M, Olivo S, DeAssis S, Gustafsson JA, Khan G, Hilakivi-Clarke L. Prepubertal estradiol and genistein exposures up-regulate BRCA1 mRNA and reduce mammary tumorigenesis. *Carcinogenesis* 25(5):741-8, 2004.

[145] Suba Zs. Beneficial role of estrogen signaling in glucose homeostasis and energy expenditure. Ch. 6. In: Johnson CC and Williams DB. eds: Glucose Uptake: Regulation, Signaling Pathways and Health Implications. Nova Science Publishers Inc. New York, 2013.

[146] Bordeleau L, Lipscombe L, Lubinski J, Ghadirian P, Foulkes WD, Neuhausen S, Ainsworth P, Pollak M, Sun P, Narod SA; Hereditary Breast Cancer Clinical Study Group. Diabetes and breast cancer among women with BRCA1 and BRCA2 mutations. *Cancer* 117(9):1812-8, 2011.

[147] Kotsopoulos J, Olopado OI, Ghadirian P, Lubinski J, Lynch HT, Isaacs C, Weber B, Kim-Sing C, Ainsworth P, Foulkes WD, Eisen A, Sun P, Narod SA. Changes in body weight and the risk of breast cancer in BRCA1 and BRCA2 mutation carriers. *Breast Cancer Res.* 7(5):R833-43, 2005.

Bibliography

Anaesthesia for patients with
endocrine disease LCCN:
2010011179 Type of material:
Book Main title: Anaesthesia for
patients with endocrine disease /
edited by M.F.M. James.
Published/Created: Oxford
[England]; New York: Oxford
University Press, 2010.
Description: xii, 266 p.: ill.
(some col.); 26 cm. ISBN:
9780199570256 (alk. paper)
0199570256 (alk. paper) LC
classification: RD599 .A53 2010
Related names: James, Michael
F. M. Contents: Basic endocrine
concepts in health and critical
illness / Naomi Levitt, Ian Ross,
and Joel Dave -- The pituitary
gland / Jeffrey J. Pasternak --
Diabetes mellitus: glucose
control: what benefit, what cost
in surgical patients? / John W.
Sear -- The thyroid gland /
M.F.M. James and P.A. Farling -
- Parathyroid disease / Philipp

Riss, Eva Schaden, and
Christian K. Spiss -- Anaesthetic
management of patients with
carcinoid tumours / Anis S.
Baraka -- Adrenal cortex / W.J.
Russell and M.F.M. James --
Adrenal medulla: the anaesthetic
management of
phaeochromocytoma / M.F.M.
James -- Endocrine emergencies
/ P.A. Farling and J.A.
Silversides -- Hormones as
pharmaceutical agents: focus on
steroids and vasopressin / John
G.T. Augoustides, Insung
Chung, and Prakash Patel --
Endocrine surgery: a personal
view / Tom R. Kurzawinski.
Subjects: Endocrine glands--
Surgery--Complications.
Anesthesia. Anesthesia--
methods. Endocrine System
Diseases--surgery. Endocrine
System Diseases--complications.
Endocrine System Diseases--
physiopathology. Notes:

Includes bibliographical references and index. Dewey class no.: 617.9/6744 NLM class no.: 2010 H-740 WK 148 A532 2010 National bib no.: GBB030264 National bib agency no.: 101526688 015493922 Other system no.: (OCoLC)ocn528397508 CALL NUMBER: RD599 .A53 2010 Copy 1 CALL NUMBER: RD599 .A53 2010 Copy 2

Canine and feline anesthesia and co-existing disease LCCN: 2014025602 Type of material: Book Main title: Canine and feline anesthesia and co-existing disease / editors, Lindsey B.C. Snyder and Rebecca A. Johnson. Published/Produced: Ames, Iowa: John Wiley & Sons Inc., 2015. Projected pub date: 1501 Description: p.; cm. ISBN: 9781118288207 (pbk.) LC classification: SF914 Related names: Snyder, Lindsey B. C., editor. Johnson, Rebecca A. (Rebecca Ann), editor. Contents: Cardiovascular disease / Jonathan M. Congdon -- Respiratory disease / David B. Brunson and Rebecca A. Johnson -- Neurologic disease / Erin Wendt-Hornickle -- Hepatobiliary disease / Carrie A. Schroeder -- Gastrointestinal disease / Juliana Peboni Figueiredo and Todd A. Green -- Renal disease / Carrie A. Schroeder -- Perioperative fluid, electrolyte, and acid-base disorders / Carolyn l. Kerr -- Endocrine disease / Berit l. Fischer -- Nutritional disease / Lindsey B.C. Snyder -- Ophthalmic disease / Phillip Lerche -- Oral and maxillofacial disorders / Christopher J. Snyder and Jason W. Soukup -- Hematologic disorders / Molly Shepard and Benjamin Brainard -- Skin and musculoskeletal diseases / Paulo V.M. Steagall -- Infectious disease / Jusmeen Sarkar -- Neoplastic disease / Veronica Salazar -- Cesarean section and pregnancy / Turi K. Aarnes and Richard M. Bednarski -- Neonatal, pediatric and geriatric concerns / Anderson Fávaro da Cunha -- Disorders related to trauma / Andre Shih. Subjects: Anesthesia--veterinary. Cat Diseases--surgery. Dog Diseases--surgery. Notes: Includes bibliographical references and index. Additional formats: Online version: Canine and feline anesthesia and co-existing disease Ames, Iowa: John Wiley & Sons Inc., 2015 9781118391594 (DLC) 2014027262 Dewey class no.: 636.089/796 NLM class no.: SF 914 Other system no.: (DNLM)

Endocrinology in clinical practice
LCCN: 2014014205 Type of
material: Book Main title:
Endocrinology in clinical
practice / editors, Philip E.
Harris and Pierre-Marc G.
Bouloux. Edition: Second
edition. Published/Produced:
Boca Raton: Taylor & Francis,
2014. Projected pub date: 1404
Description: p.; cm. ISBN:
9781841849515 (hbk.: alk.
paper) LC classification: RC648
Related names: Harris, Philip E.,
1954- editor. Bouloux, Pierre-M.
G., editor. Summary: "The
objective of the first edition was
to provide cutting-edge
information on clinical practice
for practicing endocrinologists
and doctors training in
endocrinology. The second
edition retains this ethos, but it
has been extensively updated
and modified. Endocrinology is
moving toward an increasingly
personalized approach to patient
management. This is reflected
by the increased focus on
mechanisms of disease and
biomarkers"--Provided by
publisher. Contents:
Neuroendocrine disease / Philip
E. Harris -- Familial isolated
pituitary adenomas / Vladimir
Vasilev, Renata S. Auriemma,
Adrian F. Daly, Albert Beckers -
- Surgical management of
pituitary adenomas / Garni

Barkhoudarian, Edward R.
Laws, Jr. -- Pituitary
radiotherapy / Thankamma
Ajithkumar, Michael Brada --
Replacement therapy in adult
hypopituitarism / Anna G.
Nilsson, Gudmundur Johannsson
-- IGF-I as a metabolic hormone
/ David R. Clemmons --
Radionuclide scanning in the
diagnosis and treatment of
endocrine disorders / Rakesh
Sajjan, Jamshed Bomanji --
Gastroenteropancreatic
neuroendocrine tumors
(neoplasms) / Maxime Palazzo,
Philippe Ruszniewski, Dermot
O'Toole -- Hereditary primary
hyperparathyroidism and
multiple endocrine neoplasia /
Emma Tham, Catharina Larsson
-- Coincidental adrenal masses
and adrenal cancer / Marinella
Tzanela, Dimitra Argyro
Vassiliadi, Stylianos Tsagarakis
-- Disorders of calcium
regulation / Dolores Shoback --
Metabolic bone disease / Philip
E. Harris, Pierre-Marc G.
Bouloux -- Autoimmune
endocrine disease / Terry J.
Smith, Laszlo Hegedüs --
Nonautoimmune thyroid disease
/ Arie Berghout, Alex F. Muller,
Philip E. Harris -- Differentiated
and undifferentiated thyroid
cancer / Michael J. Stechman,
David Scott-Coombes -- The
inherited basis of

hypogonadotropic hypogonadism / Pierre-Marc G. Bouloux -- Hypogonadism, erectile dysfunction, and infertility in men / Pierre-Marc G. Bouloux, Shalender Bhasin -- Amenorrhea and hirsutism / Stephen Franks -- Endocrine problems in pregnancy / Anjali Amin, Stephen Robinson -- Fluid and electrolyte disorders / Ploutarchos Tzoulis, Pierre-Marc G. Bouloux -- Endocrine hypertension / Frances McManus, John M. Connell, Marie Freel -- Obesity / Ahmed Yousseif, Efthimia Karra, Sofia Rahman, Rachel L. Batterham -- Endocrinology of aging / Prasanth N. Surampudi, Christina Wang, Yanhe Lue, Ronald Swerdloff -- Endocrine emergencies / Simon Aylwin, Ben Whitelaw. Subjects: Endocrine System Diseases--therapy. Endocrine Glands--physiopathology. Endocrine System Diseases--physiopathology. Notes: Includes bibliographical references and index. Dewey class no.: 616.4 NLM class no.: WK 140 Other system no.: (DNLM)101630068 Content type: text Media type: unmediated Carrier type: volume

Essentials of Kumar & Clark's clinical medicine LCCN:

2010026008 Type of material: Book Personal name: Ballinger, Anne. Main title: Essentials of Kumar & Clark's clinical medicine / Anne Ballinger. Edition: 5th ed. Published/Created: Edinburgh; New York: Saunders, 2012. Description: xxiii, 869 p.: col. ill.; 19 cm. ISBN: 9780702035234 0702035238 9780702035241 (International) 0702035246 (International) LC classification: RC55 .B25 2012 Other title: Essentials of Kumar and Clark's clinical medicine Contents: Ethics and communication -- Infectious diseases -- Gastroenterology and nutrition -- Liver, biliary tract, and pancreatic disease -- Haematological disease -- Malignant disease -- Rheumatology -- Water, electrolytes, and acid-base balance -- Renal disease -- Cardiovascular disease -- Respiratory disease -- Intensive care medicine -- Drug therapy, poisoning, and alcohol misuse -- Endocrine disease -- Diabetes mellitus and other disorders of metabolism -- The special senses -- Neurology -- Dermatology. Subjects: Clinical medicine--Handbooks, manuals, etc. Clinical Medicine--Handbooks. Notes: Includes index. Dewey class no.: 616 NLM class no.:

Feline emergency and critical care medicine LCCN: 2009049306 Type of material: Book Main title: Feline emergency and critical care medicine / edited by Kenneth J. Drobatz, Merilee F. Costello. Published/Created: Ames, Iowa: Wiley-Blackwell, 2010. Description: xv, 656 p.: ill. (chiefly col.); 25 cm. ISBN: 9780813823119 (pbk.: alk. paper) 0813823110 (pbk.: alk. paper) LC classification: SF985 .F415 2010 Cover title: Feline emergency & critical care medicine Related names: Drobatz, Kenneth J. Costello, Merilee F. Summary: "Until now, emergency and critical care medicine for cats has been covered only in multi-species books. Feline Emergency and Critical Care Medicine is the first book to focus solely on feline-specific emergency and critical care. Given the unique aspects of feline health and the growing interest in the specialty of feline medicine, this book serves as an essential resource for both feline-only and small animal clinicians. Designed as a quick-access manual of emergency and critical care procedures exclusively for feline patients, information is presented in an easy-to-follow outline format. Each chapter includes an algorithm of the general approach to the given condition, with helpful cross-references to the appropriate outline sections where more extensive information can be found. Pathophysiology is discussed only in enough depth to provide the clinician with adequate information to understand the clinical principles of each disease and condition. Also included as an appendix is information on emergency drugs, dosages, and indications"--Provided by publisher. Contents: Approach to the critically ill cat / Kenneth J. Drobatz -- Cardiopulmonary-cerebral resuscitation (CPCR) / Sean D. Smarick -- Shock / Merilee F. Costello -- Trauma / Erica L. Reineke -- Guidelines for anesthesia in critically ill feline patients / Lynne I Kushner -- Anesthetic protocols for systemically healthy cats / Lynne I. Kushner -- Pain management in critically ill feline patients / Lynne I. Kushner -- Fluid therapy / Garret Pachtinger -- Nutritional support for the critically ill feline patient

/ Daniel L. Chan -- Respiratory emergencies and pleural space disease / Amy V. Trow, Elizabeth Rozanski, and Armelle de Laforcade -- Upper airway disease / April L. Paul and Elizabeth Rozanski -- Lower airway disease / Benjamin M. Brainard and Lesley G. King -- Parenchymal disease / Deborah Silverstein -- General approach and overview of cardiac emergencies / Manuel Boller -- Management of specific cardiac diseases / Mark A. Oyama -- Management of thromboembolic disease secondary to heart disease / Amy J. Alwood -- Management of life-threatening arrhythmias / Meg M. Sleeper -- Less-common cardiac conditions: heartworm, syncope, pericardial disease, bacterial endocarditis, and digitalis toxicity / Jamie M. Burkitt -- Diagnostic evaluation of gastrointestinal conditions / Daniel Z. Hume -- General approach to the acute abdomen / Sara Snow and Matthew W. Beal -- Management of specific gastrointestinal conditions / Anne Marie Corrigan and Douglass K. Macintire -- Diagnostic evaluation, monitoring, and therapeutic techniques for the urologic system / Simon W. Tappin and Andrew J. Brown -- Urologic emergencies: ureter, bladder, urethra, GN, and CRF / Annie Malouin -- Acute intrinsic renal failure / Cathy Langston -- General approach and overview of the neurologic cat / Daniel J. Fletcher -- Neurologic emergencies: brain / Jessica M. Snyder -- Neurologic emergencies: spinal cord / Jessica M. Snyder -- Neurologic emergencies: peripheral / Jessica M. Snyder -- Hematologic emergencies: bleeding / Susan G. Hackner -- Hematologic emergencies: anemia / Susan G. Hackner -- Management of specific endocrine and metabolic diseases: diabets / Tara K. Trotman -- Management of specific endocrine and metabolic diseases: other / Cynthia R. Ward -- Diagnostic testing of endocrine disease in the cat / Jennifer E. Prittie -- Electrolyte disorders / Linda G. Martin and Amanda E. Veatch -- Reproductive emergencies / Page E. Yaxley and L. Ari Jutkowitz -- Pediatric emergencies / Maureen McMichael -- Ocular emergencies / Deborah C. Mandell -- Dermatologic emergencies / Jill L. Abraham -- Toxicological emergencies / Robert H. Poppenga -- Environmental emergencies / Lori S. Waddell and Elise

Mittleman Boller. Subjects: Cats--Wounds and injuries--Treatment--Handbooks, manuals, etc. Cats--Diseases--Treatment--Handbooks, manuals, etc. Veterinary emergencies--Handbooks, manuals, etc. Veterinary critical care--Handbooks, manuals, etc. Cat Diseases--therapy. Critical Care--methods. Emergencies--veterinary. Emergency Treatment--veterinary. Notes: Includes bibliographical references and index. Dewey class no.: 636.8/0896025 NLM class no.: 2010 I-813 SF 985 F3142 2010 NAL class no.: SF985 .F452 2010 National bib agency no.: 101520069 Other system no.: (OCoLC)ocn472720530 CALL NUMBER: SF985 .F415 2010 Copy 1

First aid for the anesthesiology boards LCCN: 2010015100 Type of material: Book Personal name: Bhatt, Himani. Main title: First aid for the anesthesiology boards / Himani Bhatt, Karlyn J. Powell, Dominique Aimee Jean. Published/Created: New York: McGraw-Hill Medical Pub. Division, c2010. Projected pub date: 1007 Description: p.; cm. ISBN: 9780071471787 (pbk.: alk. paper) 0071471782 (pbk.: alk. paper) LC classification:

RD82.3 .B45 2010 Related names: Powell, Karlyn J. Jean, Dominique Aimee. Contents: Machine generated contents note: Introduction: Guide to the ABA Examination -- Section 1: The Fundamentals of Anesthetic Management -- 1. Anesthetic Pharmacology -- 2. Physiology and Anesthesia -- 3. Preoperative Evaluation -- 4. The Anesthesia Machine -- 5. Monitoring and Equipment -- 6. Techniques for General Anesthesia -- 7. Techniques for Regional Anesthesia -- 8. Post-operative Recovery -- Section 2: Anesthesia for the Subspecialties -- 9. Pediatric Anesthesia -- 10. Obstetric Anesthesia -- 11. Cardiac Anesthesia -- 12. Thoracic Anesthesia -- 13. Anesthesia for Vascular Surgery -- 14. Neurosurgical Anesthesia -- 15. Anesthesia for Trauma -- 16. Critical Care -- 17. Pain Management -- 18. Anesthesia for Ophthalmic and ENT Surgeries -- 19. Anesthesia for Genitourinary Surgery -- 20. Anesthesia for Patients with Liver Disease -- 21. Anesthesia for Patients with Endocrine Disease -- 22. Anesthesia for Organ Transplantation -- 23. Anesthesia for Laparoscopic Surgery -- 24. Anesthesia for Orthopaedic Surgery -- 25. Anesthesia Outside of the

Operating Room -- 26. Special Considerations in Anesthesia Practice -- Section 3: Resuscitation Algorithms -- Section 4: Common Oral Board Topics. Subjects: Anesthesiology--Examinations, questions, etc. Anesthesia--Outlines. Notes: Includes index. Dewey class no.: 617.9/6076 NLM class no.: WO 218.2 B575f 2010 Other system no.: (DNLM)101528274

Handbook of clinical anesthesia procedures of the Massachusetts General Hospital. LCCN: 2010000516 Type of material: Book Main title: Handbook of clinical anesthesia procedures of the Massachusetts General Hospital. Edition: 8th ed. / senior editor, Wilton C. Levine; associate editors, Rae M. Allain ... [et al.]. Published/Created: Philadelphia: Wolters Kluwer Health/Lippincott Williams & Wilkins, c2010. Description: xix, 704 p.: ill.; 20 cm. Links: Publisher description http://www.loc.gov/catdir/enhan cements/fy1101/2010000516-d.html Table of contents only http://www.loc.gov/catdir/enhan cements/fy1101/2010000516-t.html ISBN: 9781605474601 1605474606 LC classification: RD82.2 .C54 2010 Cover title: Clinical anesthesia procedures of

the Massachusetts General Hospital Related names: Levine, Wilton C. Massachusetts General Hospital. Department of Anesthesia and Critical Care. Contents: Part I: Evaluating the patient before anesthesia -- Evaluating the patient before anesthesia / Alla Tauber and Mary Kraft -- Specific considerations with cardiac disease / Shahzad Shaefi and Hovig V. Chitilian -- Specific considerations with pulmonary disease / Stephanie C. Cintora and Kenneth E. Shepherd -- Specific considerations with renal disease / Rafael Vazquez and William Benedetto -- Specific considerations with liver disease / Salomon M. Maya and Wilton C. Levine -- Specific considerations with endocrine disease / Anne M. Drewry, Robert A. Peterfreund, and Stephanie L. Lee -- Infectious diseases and infection control in anesthesia / Shahzad Shaefi and Ulrich Schmidt -- Part II: Administration of anesthesia -- Safety in anesthesia / Sara N. Goldhaber-Fiebert and Jeffrey B. Cooper -- The anesthesia machine / Andrew R. Vaclavik and Greg Ginsburg -- Monitoring / Jennifer Chatburn and Warren S. Sandberg -- Intravenous and inhalation anesthetics / Claudia Benkwitz and Ken Solt -- Neuromuscular blockade / Oleg V. Evgenov and Peter F. Dunn -- Airway evaluation and management / Cosmin Gauran and Peter F. Dunn -- Administration of general anesthesia / Victor A. Chin and Stuart A. Forman -- Local anesthetics / Maryam Jowza and Rebecca D. Minehart -- Spinal, epidural, and caudal anesthesia / Jason M. Lewis and May C. M. Pian-Smith -- Regional anesthesia / Keith Fragoza and Lisa Warren -- Intra-anesthetic problems / Jonathan D. Bloom and Keith Baker -- Perioperative hemodynamic control / Brian T. Bateman and Vilma E. Ortiz -- Anesthesia for abdominal surgery / Emily A. Singer and John J. A. Marota -- Anesthesia for thoracic surgery / Junichi Naganuma and Paul H. Alfille -- Anesthesia for vascular surgery / M. Richard Pavao and Edward A. Bittner -- Anesthesia for cardiac surgery / Ethan Small and Jason Zhensheng Qu -- Anesthesia for neurosurgery / Scott A. LeGrand and Michele Szabo -- Anesthesia for head and neck surgery / Brian D. Cauley and Deborah S. Pederson -- Anesthesia for urologic surgery / Kris C. Lukauskis and William R. Kimball -- Anesthesia for geriatric patients / Zhongcong Xie and Christine Finer -- Anesthesia for surgical emergencies in the neonate / James Y. Ko ... [et al.] -- Anesthesia for pediatric surgery / Susan A. Vassallo and LIsbeth L. Pappas -- Anesthesia for obstetrics and gynecology / Amy Ortman and Lisa Leffert -- Ambulatory anesthesia / Christopher J. Hodge and LIsa Wollman -- Anesthesia outside of the operating room / Thomas J. Graetz and John J. A. Marota -- Anesthesia for trauma and burns / Vikram Kumar and Keith Baker -- Transfusion therapy / Shubha V. Y. Raju and Jonathan E. Charnin -- Part III: Perioperative issues -- The postanesthesia care unit / Asheesh Kumar and Edward E. George -- Perioperative respiratory failure / Michael R. Shaughnessy and Luca M. Bigatello -- Adult, pediatric, and newborn resuscitation / Richard M. Pino, Bradley E. Randel, and Arthur J. Tokarcyzk -- Pain / Karsten Bartels and James P. Rathmell -- Complementary and alternative medicine / Margaret A. Gargarian and P. Grace Harrell -- Ethical and end-of-life issues / Sheri Berg and Rae M. Allain -- Appendix A: supplemental drug information / Bishr Haydar. Subjects: Anesthesiology--Handbooks, manuals, etc. Anesthesia--methods--Handbooks. Anesthetics--administration & dosage--Handbooks. Perioperative Care--methods--Handbooks. Notes: Rev. ed. of: Clinical anesthesia procedures of the Massachusetts General Hospital. 7th ed. 2007. Includes bibliographical references and index. Dewey class no.: 617.9/6 NLM class no.: 2010 H-847 WO 231 C641 2010 National bib no.: GBB037529 National bib agency no.: 101522240 015505836 Other system no.: (OCoLC)ocn498974946 CALL NUMBER: RD82.2 .C54 2010 Copy 1

Harper's textbook of pediatric dermatology LCCN: 2011008692 Type of material: Book Main title: Harper's textbook of pediatric dermatology / edited by Alan Irvine, Peter Hoeger, Albert Yan. Edition: 3rd ed. Published/Created: Chichester, West Sussex, UK: Wiley-Blackwell, 2011. Projected pub date: 1105 Description: p.; cm. ISBN: 9781405176958 (hardback: alk. paper) LC classification: RJ511 .T492 2011 Portion of title: Textbook of pediatric dermatology Related names: Irvine, Alan, MD. Hoeger, Peter. Yan, Albert C.

Summary: "The third edition of this highly regarded text continues to provide a comprehensive resource for pediatric dermatologists. The book offers evidence-based diagnosis and treatment recommendations and covers both common and rare conditions, including emerging conditions and research, especially at the genetic level. A refreshing new text design makes the book more accessible, and new editors and contributors bring a distinctly international perspective to the work"--Provided by publisher. Contents: Machine generated contents note: Pyodermas and Toxin-mediated Syndromes. Skin Manifestations of Meningococcal Infection. Pitted Keratolysis, Erythrasma and Erysipeloid. Mycobacterial Infections of the Skin. Bartonella Infections: Bacillary Angiomatosis, Cat Scratch Disease and Bartonellosis. Lyme Disease. Endemic Treponematoses: Yaws, Pinta and Endemic Syphilis. Rocky Mountain Spotted Fever and Other Rickettsial Infections. Superficial Fungal Infections. Deep Mycoses. Opportunistic Infections/infections in immunocompromised. Skin Manifestations of Nutritional

Disorders. Tropical Ulcer.
Leishmaniasis. Cutaneous Larva
Migrans. Myiasis. Leprosy.
Papular Urticaria. Scabies and
Lice. Other Noxious and
Venomous Creatures. Urticaria.
Mastocytosis. Annular
Erythemas. Erythema Nodosum
and Other Forms of Panniculitis.
Erythema Multiforme, Stevens-
Johnson Syndrome and Toxic
Epidermal Necrolysis. Acne.
Psoriasis. Psoriasis -
Pathogenesis. Psoriasis -
Treatments. Pityriasis Rubra
Pilaris. Pityriasis Rosea. Lichen
Planus and Lichen Nitidus.
Lichen Striatus. Differential
Diagnosis of Vesiculobullous
Lesions. Infantile
Acropustulosis. Chronic Bullous
Disease of Childhood: Linear
IgA Disease of Childhood and
Mixed Immunobullous Disease.
Dermatitis Herpetiformis.
Pemphigus, Pemphigoid and
Epidermolysis Bullosa
Acquisita. Differential Diagnosis
of Skin Nodules and Cysts.
Granuloma Annulare. Adnexal
Disorders. Calcification and
Ossification in the Skin.
Knuckle Pads. Fibromatoses,
Hyalinoses and Stiff Skin
Syndrome. Angiolymphoid
Hyperplasia with Eosinophilia.
Skin Malignancies. Pityriasis
Lichenoides. Lymphomatoid
Papulosis. Jessner's

Lymphocytic Infiltrate of the
Skin. Cutaneous lymphomas.
The Histiocytoses, Langerhans
Cell and Non-Langerhans Cell
Histiocytosis. Disorders of
Hypopigmentation and
Hyperpigmentation. Vitiligo.
The Idiopathic Photodermatoses.
Porphyrias. Photoprotection.
Melanocytic Naevi and
Melanoma. Epidermal
Naevi/Epidermal
NaevusSyndromes. Proteus
Syndrome. Vascular
Malformations. Infantile
Haemangiomas and Other
Vascular Tumours. Disorders of
Lymphatics. Principles of
Genetics, Mosaicism and
Molecular Biology.
Chromosome Disorders. Review
of Keratin Disorders.
Epidermolysis Bullosa. Kindler
syndrome. Generalized
Disorders of Cornification (the
Ichthyoses). Netherton's
Syndrome. Palmoplantar
Keratodermas. Keratosis Pilaris.
The Erythrokeratodermas.
Darier's Disease. The
Porokeratoses. Ectodermal
Dysplasias. The
Neurofibromatoses. Tuberous
Sclerosis. Incontinentia
Pigmenti. Pigmentary
Mosaicism (Ito syndrome). The
Gorlin (Naevoid Basal Cell
Carcinoma) Syndrome. Focal
Dermal Hypoplasia Syndrome

(Synonym: Goltz Syndrome). Premature Ageing Syndromes (Laminopathies). Xeroderma Pigmentosum, Cockayne's Syndrome and Trichothiodystrophy. Rothmund-Thomson Syndrome. Bloom's Syndrome, Dyskeratosis Congenita and Fanconi's Syndrome. Genetic Diseases that Predispose to Malignancy. Dyschromatoses. Prenatal Diagnosis of Inherited Skin Disorders. Skin Gene Therapy. Disorders of Fat Tissue. Ehlers-Danlos Syndromes. Cutis Laxa. Pseudoxanthoma Elasticum. Buschke-Ollendorff Syndrome, Marfan's Syndrome, Osteogenesis Imperfecta, Anetodermas and Atrophodermas. Striae. Diseases of the Oral Mucosa and Tongue. Hair Disorders. Alopecia Areata. Nail Disorders. Genital Disease in Children. Vulvovaginitis and Lichen Sclerosus. Sexually Transmitted Diseases in Children and Adolescents. Non-Accidental injury and mimickers. Physical and Sexual Abuse and mimickers. Neutrophilic disorders. Crohn's Disease and Granulomatous Cheilitis (OFG). Sarcoidosis. Amyloidosis. Henoch-Schönlein Purpura. Acute Haemorrhagic Oedema of the Skin in Infancy.

Purpura Fulminans. Urticarial Vasculitis. Erythema Elevatum Diutinum. Pigmented Purpuras. Erythromelalgia. Wegener's Granulomatosis, Polyarteritis Nodosa, Behçet's Disease and Relapsing Polychondritis. Kawasaki Disease. Inherited Metabolic Disorders and the Skin. Cystic Fibrosis. Carotenaemia. Cutaneous Manifestations of Endocrine Disease. Morphoea (Synonym: Localized Scleroderma). Systemic Sclerosis in Childhood. Juvenile Idiopathic Arthritis, Systemic Lupus Erythematosus and Dermatomyositis. Recurrent Fever Syndromes. Immunodeficiency Syndromes. Graft-Versus-Host Disease. Coping with Chronic Skin Disease. Physiological Habits, Self-mutilation and Factitious Disorders. Principles of Paediatric Dermatological Therapy. Use of emerging biologic treatments in children. Hypersensitivity Reactions To Drugs. Poisoning and Paediatric Skin. Basic Skin Surgery Techniques. More Complex Skin Surgery. Laser Treatment for Cutaneous Vascular Anomalies. The Use of Resurfacing, Pigment and Depilation Lasers in Children. Sedation and Anaesthesia.

Nursing Care of Paediatric Skin. Subjects: Pediatric dermatology. Skin--Diseases. Skin Diseases. Child. Infant. Notes: Rev. ed. of: Textbook of pediatric dermatology / edited by John Harper, Arnold Oranje, Neil Prose. 2nd ed. 2006. Includes bibliographical references and index. Dewey class no.: 618.92/5 NLM class no.: WS 260 Other system no.: (DNLM)101554851

Medical nutrition and disease: a case-based approach LCCN: 2014019651 Type of material: Book Main title: Medical nutrition and disease: a case-based approach / editor-in-chief, Lisa Hark, Darwin Deen, Gail Morrison. Edition: Fifth edition. Published/Produced: Chichester, West Sussex, UK; Hoboken, NJ: John Wiley & Sons Inc., 2014. Projected pub date: 1411 Description: p.; cm. ISBN: 9781118652435 (pbk.) Related names: Hark, Lisa, editor. Deen, Darwin, editor. Morrison, Gail, editor. Contents: Overview of nutrition assessment in clinical care / Lisa Hark, Darwin Deen, and Alix Pruzansky -- Vitamins, minerals, and dietary supplements / Kelly Keenan, Herbert Hodgson, and Darwin Deen -- Nutrition in pregnancy and lactation / Elizabeth Horwitz

West, Lisa Hark, and Darwin Deen -- Infants, children, and adolescents / Carine M. Lenders, Kathy Ireland, and Andrew M. Tershakovec -- Older adults / Cecilia Borden and Lisa Hark -- Cardiovascular disease / Jo Ann S. Carson and Scott M. Grundy -- Gastrointestinal disease / Julie Vanderpool and Charles Vanderpool-- Endocrine disease: diabetes mellitus / Marion J. Franz -- Pulmonary disease / Horace M. DeLisser, Bianca Collymore, and Calvin Lambert -- Renal disease / Jean Stover, Gail Morrison, and Susan Lupackino -- Cancer prevention and treatment / Tamara B. Kaplan, Monica H. Crawford, and Pranay Soni -- Enteral nutrition support / Jill Murphree and Douglas Seidner -- Parenteral nutrition support / Laura Matarese, Ezra Steiger, and Monica Habib. Subjects: Diet Therapy--Case Reports. Nutritional Physiological Phenomena--Case Reports. Nutritional Support--Case Reports. Notes: Includes bibliographical references and index. Additional formats: Online version: Medical nutrition and disease Fifth edition. Chichester, West Sussex, UK; Hoboken, NJ: John Wiley & Sons Inc., 2014 9781118652411 (DLC)

2014020672 Dewey class no.: RM216 613.2 NLM class no.: WB 400 Other system no.: (DNLM)101632903

Medical-surgical nursing test success: an unfolding case study review LCCN: 2013004101 Type of material: Book Personal name: Gittings, Karen K. Main title: Medical-surgical nursing test success: an unfolding case study review / Karen K. Gittings, Rhonda M. Brogdon, Frances H. Cornelius. Published/Created: New York, NY: Springer Pub., c2013. Description: xiii, 317 p.; 26 cm. ISBN: 9780826195760 (pbk.) 0826195768 (pbk.) 9780826195777 (e-book) LC classification: RT55 .G53 2013 Related names: Brogdon, Rhonda M. Cornelius, Frances H. Contents: Nursing care of the patient with cardiovascular disease -- Nursing care of the patient with pulmonary disease -- Nursing care of the patient with renal disease -- Nursing care of the patient with gastrointestinal disease -- Nursing care of the patient with neurological disease -- Nursing care of the patient with endocrine disease -- Nursing care of the patient with immunological disease -- Nursing care of the patient with hematological disease -- Nursing care of the patient with musculoskeletal disease -- Nursing care of the patient with infectious diseases. Subjects: Nursing Care--methods--Problems and Exercises. Nursing Assessment--methods--Problems and Exercises. Perioperative Nursing--methods--Problems and Exercises. Notes: Includes bibliographical references and index. Dewey class no.: 610.73076 NLM class no.: WY 18.2 Other system no.: (DNLM)101601172 Shelf Location: FLM2014 020561 CALL NUMBER: RT55 .G53 2013 OVERFLOWA5S

Motivational interviewing in nursing practice: empowering the patient LCCN: 2009038826 Type of material: Book Personal name: Dart, Michelle A. Main title: Motivational interviewing in nursing practice: empowering the patient / Michelle A. Dart. Published/Created: Sudbury, Mass.: Jones and Bartlett Publishers, c2011. Description: viii, 289 p.: ill.; 23 cm. ISBN: 9780763773854 (alk. paper) 0763773859 (alk. paper) LC classification: RT86.3 .D37 2011 Contents: Basics of motivational interviewing -- Making the pieces fit: therapeutic communication and the nursing process -- Motivational interviewing as evidence-based practice -- Challenges in motivational interviewing -- Developmental considerations -- Motivational interviewing in cardiac health -- Motivational interviewing in endocrine disease -- Motivational interviewing in digestive health -- Motivational interviewing in genitourinary health -- Motivational interviewing in neurological disorders -- Motivational interviewing in musculoskeletal disorders -- Motivational interviewing in mental health disorders -- Motivational interviewing in pulmonary disorders -- Motivational interviewing in preventive care -- Future of motivational interviewing in nursing practice. Subjects: Nurse and patient. Motivational interviewing. Counseling--methods. Health Promotion--methods. Motivation. Patient Education as Topic--methods. Notes: Includes bibliographical references and index. Dewey class no.: 610.7306/99 NLM class no.: 2010 E-240 WY 87 D226m 2011 National bib agency no.: 101515409 Other system no.: (OCoLC)ocn439472122 CALL NUMBER: RT86.3 .D37 2011

Pre-operative management of the patient with chronic disease LCCN: 2013444414 Type of material: Book Main title: Pre-operative management of the patient with chronic disease / editors, Ansgar M. Brambrink, Peter Rock, Jeffrey R. Kirsch. Published/Created: Philadelphia, Pa.: Elsevier, 2013. Description: xvii, [993]-1230 p.: ill. (some col.); 24 cm. ISBN: 9780323242295 0323242294 LC classification: RA973.5 .P74 2013 Related names: Brambrink, Ansgar. Rock, Peter. Kirsch, Jeffrey R., 1957- Contents: Preface: Pre-operative management of the patient with chronic disease / Ansgar M. Brambrink, Peter Rock, and Jeffrey R. Kirsch -- Patients with disease of brain, cerebral vasculature, and spine / Joshua W. Sappenfield and Douglas G. Martz Jr -- Patients with neuromuscular disorder / Palak Turakhia, Brian Barrick, and Jeffrey Berman -- Patients with ischemic heart disease / Patrick N. Odonkor and Alina M. Grigore -- Patients with pacemaker or implantable cardiverter-defibrillator / Peter M. Schulman, ... et al. -- Patients with vascular disease / Anne-Marie Manley and Sarah E. Reck -- Patients with chronic pulmonary disease / Caron M.

Hong and Samuel M. Galvagno Jr -- Patients with chronic kidney disease / Alicia Gruber Kalamas and Claus U. Niemann -- Patients with chronic endocrine disease / Mary Josephine Njoku -- Patients with immunodeficiency / Michael J. Hannaman and Melissa J. Ertl -- Patients with disorders of thrombosis and hemostasis / Andrea Orfanakis and Thomas DeLoughery -- Patients requiring perioperative nutritional support / T. Miko Enomoto, Dawn Larson, and Robert G. Martindale -- Patients with chronic pain / Joseph Salama-Hanna and Grace Chen. Subjects: Chronically ill--Surgery. Chronically ill--Surgery--Complications. Chronically ill--Surgery--Risk factors. Notes: "November 2013." Includes bibliographical references and index. Series: Medical clinics of North America, 0025-7125; v. 97, no. 6 Medical clinics of North America; v. 97, no. 6. Dewey class no.: 362.16 Other system no.: (OCoLC)ocn847348896 CALL NUMBER: RA973.5 .P74 2013 Copy 2 Request in: Jefferson or Adams Building Reading Rooms Shelf Location: FLM2014 017998 CALL NUMBER: RA973.5 .P74 2013 OVERFLOWA5S

Small animal pathology for veterinary technicians LCCN: 2013039731 Type of material: Book Personal name: Johnson, Amy, 1973- author. Main title: Small animal pathology for veterinary technicians / Amy Johnson, BS, CVT, RLATG. Published/Produced: Ames, Iowa: Wiley Blackwell, 2014. Description: x, 226 pages: color illustrations; 25 cm ISBN: 9781118434215 (pbk.) 1118434218 (pbk.) LC classification: SF769 .J64 2014 Contents: Canine infectious disease -- Feline infectious disease -- Rabies -- Gastrointestinal tract disease -- Urinary tract disease -- Reproductive disease -- Endocrine disease -- Ocular disease -- Integumentary diseases -- Musculoskeletal disease -- Hematologic and lymph disease -- Diseases of rabbits, guinea pigs, and chinchillas -- Diseases of ferrets -- Diseases of hamsters, gerbils, and rats. Subjects: Animals--Diseases--Handbooks, manuals, etc. Dogs--Diseases--Handbooks, manuals, etc. Cats--Diseases--Handbooks, manuals, etc. Pets--Diseases--Handbooks, manuals, etc. Animal Diseases--Handbooks. Pets--Handbooks. Animal Technicians--Handbooks. Notes: Includes bibliographical references and index. Additional formats: Online version: Johnson, Amy, 1973- author. Small animal pathology for veterinary technicians Ames, Iowa: John Wiley & Sons, 2014 9781118747254 (DLC) 2013042889 Dewey class no.: 636.089/607 NLM class no.: SF 981 Other system no.: (DNLM)101618117 Content type: text Media type: unmediated Carrier type: volume Shelf Location: FLM2014 202625 CALL NUMBER: SF769 .J64 2014 OVERFLOWA5S

The diagnosis of psychosis LCCN: 2010051717 Type of material: Book Personal name: Cardinal, Rudolf N. Main title: The diagnosis of psychosis / Rudolf N. Cardinal, Edward T. Bullmore. Published/Created: Cambridge, UK; New York: Cambridge University Press, 2011. Description: xxv, 373 p.: ill.; 24 cm. Links: Cover image http://assets.cambridge.org/9780 5211/64849/cover/97805211648 49.jpg ISBN: 9780521164849 (pbk.) 0521164842 (pbk.) LC classification: RC512 .C356 2011 Related names: Bullmore, Edward T. Summary: "Psychosis has many causes. Psychiatrists typically receive the most thorough training in its diagnosis, but the diagnosis of psychosis secondary to nonpsychiatric conditions is not often emphasized. An understanding of the underlying cause of psychosis is important for effective management. The Diagnosis of Psychosis bridges the gap between psychiatry and medicine, providing a comprehensive review of primary and secondary causes of psychosis. It covers both common and rare causes in a clinically focused guide. Useful both for teaching and reference, the text covers physical and mental state examination, describes key investigations, and summarizes the non-psychiatric features of medical conditions causing psychosis. Particularly relevant for psychiatrists and trainees in psychiatry, this volume will also assist neurologists and general physicians who encounter psychosis in their practice"-- Provided by publisher. Contents: Machine generated contents note: Abbreviations and symbols; Preface; Acknowledgements; Part I. The Causes of Psychosis: 1. Introduction; 2. Methods; 3. Delirium; 4. Neurodevelopmental disorders and chromosomal abnormalities;

5. Neurodegenerative disorders; 6. Focal neurological disease; 7. Malignancy; 8. Infectious and postinfectious syndromes; 9. Endocrine disease; 10. Inborn errors of metabolism; 11. Nutritional deficiency; 12. Other acquired metabolic disorders; 13. Autoimmune rheumatic disorders and vasculitides; 14. Other autoimmune encephalopathies; 15. Poisoning; 16. Sleep disorders; 17. Sensory deprivation and impairment; 18. Miscellaneous; 19. Catatonia; 20. Agitation and bizarre behaviour; 21. Primary psychiatric disease; 22. Factitious disorder and malingering; 23. Multiple simultaneous causes of psychosis, and questions of causality; Part II. A Clinical Approach to the Diagnosis of Psychosis: 24. History and examination; 25. Initial investigations relevant to psychosis; 26; Putting it together: clinical and paraclinical clues; 27. Further investigations relevant to psychosis; 28. Classificatory approach for psychosis of unknown aetiology; 29. Conclusion; 30. Appendices; 31. References; Index. Subjects: Psychoses--Diagnosis. Physicians (General practice) Psychotic Disorders--diagnosis. Psychotic Disorders--etiology. Notes: Includes bibliographical references (p. 289-361) and index. Series: Cambridge medicine Cambridge medicine. Dewey class no.: 616.89 NLM class no.: 2011 F-063 WM 200 Other class no.: MED102000 National bib agency no.: 101549390 Other system no.: (OCoLC)ocn671710663 CALL NUMBER: RC512 .C356 2011 Copy 1 CALL NUMBER: RC512 .C356 2011 FT MEADE Copy 2

Index

D

T

U